THE "I LOVE MY AIR FRYER"

Keto Diet 5-Ingredient

RECIPE BOOK

From *Bacon and Cheese Quiche* to *Chicken Cordon Bleu*, 175 Quick and Easy Keto Recipes

Sam Dillard of HeyKetoMama.com

Author of The *"I Love My Air Fryer"*
Keto Diet Recipe Book

Adams Media

New York London Toronto Sydney New Delhi

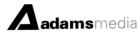

Adams Media
An Imprint of Simon & Schuster, Inc.
100 Technology Center Drive
Stoughton, MA 02072

First Adams Media trade paperback edition May 2020

ADAMS MEDIA and colophon are trademarks of Simon & Schuster.

For information about special discounts for bulk purchases, please contact Simon & Schuster Special Sales at 1-866-506-1949 or business@simonandschuster.com.

The Simon & Schuster Speakers Bureau can bring authors to your live event. For more information or to book an event contact the Simon & Schuster Speakers Bureau at 1-866-248-3049 or visit our website at www.simonspeakers.com.

Interior design by Erin Alexander
Photographs by James Stefiuk

Manufactured in the United States of America

6 2021

Library of Congress Cataloging-in-Publication Data
Names: Dillard, Sam, author.
Title: The "I love my air fryer" keto diet 5-ingredient recipe book / Sam Dillard of HeyKetoMama.com, author of The "I Love My Air Fryer" Keto Diet Recipe Book.
Description: Avon, Massachusetts: Adams Media, 2020. | Series: "I love my" series. Includes index.
Identifiers: LCCN 2019054287 | ISBN 9781507212998 (pb) | ISBN 9781507213001 (ebook)
Subjects: LCSH: Reducing diets--Recipes. | Ketogenic diet. | Hot air frying. | LCGFT: Cookbooks.
Classification: LCC RM222.2 .D5746 2020 | DDC 641.7/7--dc23
LC record available at https://lccn.loc.gov/2019054287

ISBN 978-1-5072-1299-8
ISBN 978-1-5072-1300-1 (ebook)

Contains material adapted from the following title published by Adams Media, an Imprint of Simon & Schuster, Inc.: *The "I Love My Air Fryer" Keto Diet Recipe Book* by Sam Dillard, copyright © 2019, ISBN 978-1-5072-0992-9.

Contents

Introduction

If you have an air fryer, you've already experienced the quick cooking times and ease of use that show why the demand for this revolutionary appliance is so high. If you're still on the fence about buying one, get ready to flex your culinary muscles and get excited about cooking. You'll soon be hooked and using your air fryer to prepare nearly every meal. But what's so special about air frying?

The air fryer can replace your oven, microwave, deep fryer, and dehydrator, and evenly cook delicious meals in a fraction of the time (and electricity costs) you're used to. Air frying makes it easy to feed your family healthy, irresistible meals with just five ingredients or less!

An air fryer can also help you succeed on the keto diet. Typically, fried foods are loaded with carbohydrates, so you might assume you have to avoid them altogether when on a keto diet. But when you use the air fryer, you can get the distinct crunch and mouthwatering taste of your fried favorites without the carbs. And you can choose your own low-carb breading! Another benefit to air frying is how much it shortens cooking time. This is especially crucial when you are hungry, short on time, and running low on supplies—a recipe for cheating on your diet. That's why your air fryer will be your best friend throughout your keto journey and help you stay on track, without venturing outside of a small list of ingredients and pantry staples.

Throughout this book you'll learn everything you need to know about using an air fryer, as well as some basics that will help you succeed on the ketogenic diet—plus 175 irresistible five-ingredient recipes for every occasion. Let's get air frying!

Cooking with an Air Fryer

Cooking with an air fryer is as easy as using a microwave. Anybody can do it, and after just a few uses you'll wish you had switched over to this genius method of cooking earlier. This chapter will introduce you to air-frying options and accessories to maximize your cooking time and get delicious, crispy results. It will also explain how to keep your air fryer clean and offer essentials you'll want to stock up on so that you can whip up a delicious meal with just five ingredients or less any day of the week.

While this chapter will cover the basics of air frying, the first step is reading the manual that came with your air fryer. The recent rise in popularity of the appliance means that you'll find a variety of models with different settings and sizes on the market. A thorough knowledge of how to use your specific air fryer is the key to success and will familiarize you with troubleshooting issues as well as safety functions. Read over the manual and wash all parts with warm, soapy water before first use to help you feel ready to unleash your culinary finesse.

Why Air Frying?

Air frying is increasingly popular because it allows you to quickly and evenly prepare delicious meals with little fat and little effort. Here are just a few of the reasons you'll want to switch to air frying:

- **It replaces other cooking appliances.** You can use your air fryer in place of your oven, microwave, deep fryer, and dehydrator! Using one small device, you can quickly cook up perfect dishes for every meal without sacrificing flavor.

- **It cooks faster than traditional cooking methods.** Air frying works by circulating hot air around the cooking chamber. This results in fast and even cooking, using a fraction of the energy of your oven. Most air fryers can be set to a maximum temperature of 400°F, so just about anything you can make in an oven, you can make in an air fryer.

- **It uses little to no cooking oil.** A main selling point of air fryers is that you can achieve beautifully cooked foods using little to no cooking oil. Even people following the keto diet can appreciate the lower fat content; calorie counts are important if you're following keto for weight loss, or if you track your macros and choose to use your calories otherwise.

- **Cleanup is fast.** Any method of cooking will dirty your cooker, but your air fryer's smaller cooking chamber and removable basket make thorough cleanup a breeze!

Choosing an Air Fryer

When choosing an air fryer, the two most important factors to focus on are size and temperature range. Air fryers are usually measured by quart size and range from about 1.2 quarts to 10 or more quarts. Thanks to the number of models available, you can now even find air fryer "ovens"—larger convection oven–type appliances that you can use to cook multiple racks of food at the same time. This book is based on a four-person air fryer with a 3-quart capacity and 1425 watts of power. If you're looking to cook meals to feed a family, you might be interested in at least a 5.3-quart fryer that can be used to beautifully roast an entire chicken. If your counter space is limited, and you're cooking for only one or two, you can make do with a much smaller air fryer. As for temperature range, some air fryers allow you the ability to dehydrate foods because you can cook them at a very low temperature, say 120°F, for a long period of time. Depending on the functions you need, you'll want to make sure your air fryer has the appropriate cooking capacity and temperature range.

The Functions of an Air Fryer

Most air fryers are equipped with buttons to help you prepare anything, such as grilling the perfect salmon, roasting an entire chicken, or even baking a chocolate cake.

These buttons are programmed to preset times and temperatures based on your specific air fryer. Because of the wide variety of air fryers on the market, all the recipes in this book were created using manual times and temperatures, without preheating. Every air fryer allows you to set these yourself. Still, it is important to know how the cooking programs work on your air fryer and when to use them.

Essential Accessories

Your air fryer's cooking chamber is basically just a large open space for the hot air to circulate. This is a huge advantage because it gives you the option to incorporate several different accessories into your cooking. These accessories broaden the number of recipes you can make in your air fryer and open up options you never would've thought were possible. Here are some of the common accessories.

- **Metal holder.** This circular rack is used to add a second layer to your cooking surface so you can maximize space and cook multiple things at once. It's particularly helpful when you're cooking meat and vegetables and don't want to wait for one to finish to get started on the other.

- **Skewer rack.** Similar to a metal holder, it has built-in metal skewers that make roasting kebabs a breeze.

- **Ramekins.** Small ramekins are great for making mini cakes and quiche. If they're oven safe, they're safe to use in your air fryer.

- **Cake pans.** You can find specially made cake pans for your air fryer that fit perfectly into the cooking chamber. They also come with a built-in handle so you can easily pull them out when your cakes are done baking.

- **Cupcake pan.** A cupcake pan usually comes with seven mini cups and takes up the entire chamber of a 5.3-quart air fryer.

These versatile cups are perfect for muffins, cupcakes, and even eggs. If you don't want to go this route, you can also use individual silicone baking cups.

- **Parchment paper.** Specially precut parchment paper can make cleanup even easier when baking with your air fryer. Additionally, you can find parchment paper with precut holes for easy steaming.

- **Pizza pan.** Yes, you can bake a pizza in your air fryer, and this book includes several recipes for different kinds of keto-friendly pizzas. This is a great option for easily getting the perfect shape every time.

Accessory Removal

At some point you will need to get those helpful accessories out of your air fryer without burning yourself. Here are some tools that will allow you to take items out of your appliance safely and easily.

- **Tongs.** These will be helpful when lifting meat in and out of the air fryer. Tongs are also useful for removing cooking pans that don't come with handles.

- **Oven mitts.** Sometimes simple is best. Your food will be very hot when you remove it, so it's great to have these around to protect your hands.

Cleaning Your Air Fryer

Before cleaning it, first ensure that your air fryer is completely cool and unplugged. To clean the air fryer pan you'll need to:

1. Remove the air fryer pan from the base. Fill the pan with hot water and dish soap. Let the pan soak with the frying basket inside for 10 minutes.
2. Clean the basket thoroughly with a sponge or brush.
3. Remove the fryer basket and scrub the underside and outside walls.
4. Clean the air fryer pan with a sponge or brush.
5. Let everything air-dry and return to the air fryer base.

To clean the outside of your air fryer, simply wipe with a damp cloth. Then, be sure all components are in the correct position before beginning your next cooking adventure.

What Is Keto?

The ketogenic, or keto, diet is a very low-carb, moderate-protein, high-fat diet that allows the body to fuel itself without the use of glucose or high levels of carbohydrates. When the body is in short supply of glucose, ketones are made in the liver from the breakdown of fats through a process called ketosis. (Please note this differs from ketoacidosis.) With careful tracking, creative meals, and self-control, this diet can help you lose weight, lower your blood sugar, regulate insulin levels, and control cravings.

When you eat a very high-carb diet (pizza, pasta, pastries), your body takes those carbs and turns them into glucose to power itself. When you cut out the carbs, your body burns fat instead. Typically, a ketogenic diet restricts carbs to 0–50 grams per day.

What Are Macros?

Macronutrients, or macros, are the three nutrients your body uses to produce energy. They include carbohydrates, protein, and fat. When you're following keto, it is very important to track how many grams of each macronutrient you consume each day.

- Carbs should constitute around 5 percent of your daily calories
- Protein should constitute around 25 percent of your daily calories
- Healthy fats should constitute around 70 percent of your daily calories

Some of the best-quality fats come from natural sources such as fish, avocados, and nuts. These fats can help reduce your cholesterol, keep your heart strong, and fuel your body throughout the day. You should always beware of unhealthy trans fats and saturated fats, however, which can come from foods like cookies and french fries. Overconsumption of these, especially in conjunction with a high-carb diet, can contribute to heart disease, low energy, and unwanted weight gain.

Net Carbs

Most people following keto opt to track net carbs instead of total carbs. You can figure out net carbs by subtracting your dietary fiber intake from your total carb intake:

Total carbs – dietary fiber = net carbs

You can also subtract sugar alcohols from the total carb count. Net is generally the preferred method because of how your body reacts to the fiber and sugar alcohols.

On nutrition labels, the grams of dietary fiber and sugar alcohols are included in the total carb count, but because fiber and (some) sugar alcohols are carbs that your body can't digest, they have no effect on your blood sugar levels and can be subtracted.

Tips to Remember

Keep these tips in mind as you plan your daily meals:

- **Carbs are a limit:** Don't go above your allotted daily net carbs.

- **Protein is a goal:** This is the most important macro to hit. If you're losing weight, you want to make sure you're eating enough protein to keep you from losing muscle.

- **Fat is a lever—use it to adjust your diet:** In the keto diet, fat is designed to keep you full. If you're hungry, go ahead and eat that healthy fat up to your limit. If you're not hungry, you don't have to hit your fat macros.

With the quick and easy recipes in this book, you should never feel deprived on your keto journey. Just remember, if you fall off the wagon, the most important thing is to get back on as quickly as possible. Allow yourself grace and time, but never give up just because you slipped up.

Pantry Staples

Now that you have a better understanding of your air fryer and the ketogenic diet, you're ready to get cooking...almost. Each recipe in this book has five or fewer main ingredients, but also included are some kitchen staples in addition to those five to help make sure the tastes and textures of your meals come out perfect. I've identified seven nonperishable pantry staples that you likely already have in your kitchen and that you'll want to have on hand when creating the recipes in this book:

- Salt
- Ground black pepper
- Paprika
- Garlic powder
- Baking powder
- Coconut oil
- Vanilla extract

These must-haves were chosen for their versatility and frequent use in not just the recipes that follow, but also in recipes encountered online, at family gatherings and parties, and more. In each recipe in this book, you'll find a list of which of these staples you'll also need, so be sure to stock up on anything you may be running low on beforehand.

With this final information in hand, you are truly ready to get cooking! Throughout the following chapters you'll find plenty of delicious, five-ingredient recipes to suit all tastes. Use these recipes as your guide, and always feel free to season intuitively and customize dishes to your liking—just be aware that doing so will change the provided nutritional information.

2

Breakfast

Breakfast is often referred to as the most important meal because of its role in getting your day started in the right direction. It can be tough to fit a tasty breakfast into your morning, especially when you hit the snooze button on your alarm clock one too many times or you're rushing to get the kids out the door for school. Following a keto diet can make breakfast all the more complicated, leading to the temptation to pick up something fast and unhealthy in the drive-through line.

Fortunately, this chapter is here to save your morning. You'll find lots of delicious, easy recipes to step up your keto breakfast game—with just five ingredients or less. From Blueberry Muffins to Cinnamon Rolls, you'll be fueled and focused for the day ahead without sacrificing an ounce of flavor!

Chocolate Chip Muffins

These fluffy muffins are a great way to start your day with a bit of a treat. In just minutes you'll have a crowd-pleasing, sugar-free keto breakfast without having to heat up your oven. Muffins will keep in a covered container in the refrigerator for up to 4 days.

- **Pantry Staples: Baking powder**
- **Hands-On Time: 5 minutes**
- **Cook Time: 15 minutes**

Yields 6 muffins

1½ cups blanched finely ground almond flour

⅓ cup granular brown erythritol

4 tablespoons salted butter, melted

2 large eggs, whisked

1 tablespoon baking powder

½ cup low-carb chocolate chips

1. In a large bowl, combine all ingredients. Evenly pour batter into six silicone muffin cups greased with cooking spray.

2. Place muffin cups into air fryer basket. Adjust the temperature to 320°F and set the timer for 15 minutes. Muffins will be golden brown when done.

3. Let muffins cool in cups 15 minutes to avoid crumbling. Serve warm.

PER SERVING (1 MUFFIN)

CALORIES: 329	FAT: 29g
PROTEIN: 10g	SODIUM: 328mg
FIBER: 8g	CARBOHYDRATES: 28g
NET CARBOHYDRATES: 4g	SUGAR: 1g
SUGAR ALCOHOL: 16g	

GIVE THEM YOUR OWN TWIST
Feel free to experiment with flavor extracts by adding ½ teaspoon to the batter before baking. And if you want a little crunch, adding macadamia nuts or pecans will make these fluffy muffins even more filling!

Blueberry Muffins

If you're looking for the perfect breakfast muffins made in a flash, this recipe will start your day off right. Even better, you can make them ahead of time, freeze them, and heat them up in your air fryer for 3 minutes at 350°F when you're ready to enjoy!

- **Pantry Staples: Baking powder**
- **Hands-On Time: 5 minutes**
- **Cook Time: 15 minutes**

Yields 6 muffins

1½ cups blanched finely ground almond flour

½ cup granular erythritol

4 tablespoons salted butter, melted

2 large eggs, whisked

2 teaspoons baking powder

⅓ cup fresh blueberries, chopped

1 In a large bowl, combine all ingredients. Evenly pour batter into six silicone muffin cups greased with cooking spray.

2 Place muffin cups into air fryer basket. Adjust the temperature to 320°F and set the timer for 15 minutes. Muffins should be golden brown when done.

3 Let muffins cool in cups 15 minutes to avoid crumbling. Serve warm.

PER SERVING (1 MUFFIN)

CALORIES: 269

PROTEIN: 8g

FIBER: 3g

NET CARBOHYDRATES: 4g

SUGAR ALCOHOL: 16g

FAT: 24g

SODIUM: 165mg

CARBOHYDRATES: 23g

SUGAR: 2g

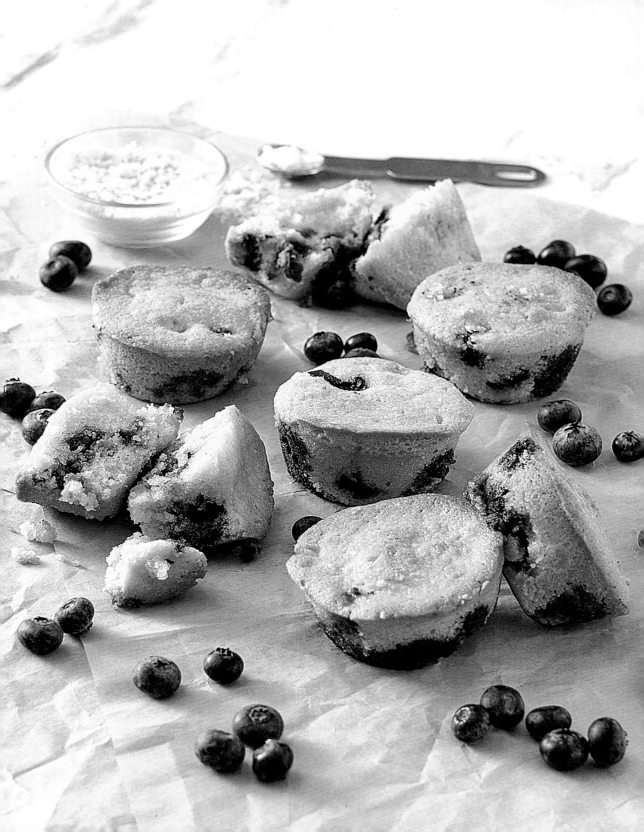

Spice Muffins

Allspice is an aromatic blend that may remind you of cloves or cinnamon. If you don't have any on hand, you can substitute an equal amount of pumpkin pie spice. This combination of fall flavors will bring an extra bit of coziness to your day, especially when served alongside a warm cup of coffee or tea.

- **Pantry Staples: Baking powder**
- **Hands-On Time: 5 minutes**
- **Cook Time: 15 minutes**

Yields 6 muffins

1 cup blanched finely ground almond flour
¼ cup granular erythritol
2 tablespoons salted butter, melted
1 large egg, whisked
2 teaspoons baking powder
1 teaspoon ground allspice

1　In a large bowl, combine all ingredients. Evenly pour batter into six silicone muffin cups greased with cooking spray.

2　Place muffin cups into air fryer basket. Adjust the temperature to 320°F and set the timer for 15 minutes. Cooked muffins should be golden brown.

3　Let muffins cool in cups 15 minutes to avoid crumbling. Serve warm.

PER SERVING (1 MUFFIN)

CALORIES: 160	**FAT:** 14g
PROTEIN: 5g	**SODIUM:** 123mg
FIBER: 2g	**CARBOHYDRATES:** 20g
NET CARBOHYDRATES: 2g	**SUGAR:** 1g
SUGAR ALCOHOL: 16g	

Bacon, Egg, and Cheese Calzones

This simple recipe is great for making ahead and taking on the go. These delicious, cheesy calzones reheat well and make for a superfilling and tasty breakfast. The keto "breading" is fluffy, which gives it that ultimate comfort-food feel.

- **Pantry Staples: None**
- **Hands-On Time: 15 minutes**
- **Cook Time: 12 minutes**

Serves 4

2 large eggs

1 cup blanched finely ground almond flour

2 cups shredded mozzarella cheese

2 ounces cream cheese, softened and broken into small pieces

4 slices cooked sugar-free bacon, crumbled

FATHEAD DOUGH

This mozzarella cheese–based dough is famous in the keto community for its breadlike qualities and extreme versatility. There are different variations, but generally it can be used for anything from a calzone to an Easy Keto Danish (see recipe in Chapter 9!). If you find that your dough is sticky, wet your hands with water before molding it.

1 Beat eggs in a small bowl. Pour into a medium nonstick skillet over medium heat and scramble. Set aside.

2 In a large microwave-safe bowl, mix flour and mozzarella. Add cream cheese to bowl.

3 Place bowl in microwave and cook 45 seconds on high to melt cheese, then stir with a fork until a soft dough ball forms.

4 Cut a piece of parchment to fit air fryer basket. Separate dough into two sections and press each out into an 8" round.

5 On half of each dough round, place half of the scrambled eggs and crumbled bacon. Fold the other side of the dough over and press to seal the edges.

6 Place calzones on ungreased parchment and into air fryer basket. Adjust the temperature to 350°F and set the timer for 12 minutes, turning calzones halfway through cooking. Crust will be golden and firm when done.

7 Let calzones cool on a cooking rack 5 minutes before serving.

PER SERVING

CALORIES: 477	**FAT:** 35g
PROTEIN: 28g	**SODIUM:** 665mg
FIBER: 3g	**CARBOHYDRATES:** 10g
NET CARBOHYDRATES: 7g	**SUGAR:** 3g

Denver Eggs

Eggs are a great source of protein, and one of the easiest bases for a hearty keto breakfast. No need to fire up the skillet for this recipe, though—all of the delicious flavors come together in minutes in your air fryer.

- **Pantry Staples: Salt, ground black pepper**
- **Hands-On Time: 5 minutes**
- **Cook Time: 15 minutes**

Serves 2

3 large eggs
1 tablespoon salted butter, melted
¼ cup seeded and chopped green bell pepper
2 tablespoons peeled and chopped yellow onion
¼ cup chopped cooked no-sugar-added ham
¼ teaspoon salt
¼ teaspoon ground black pepper

1 Crack eggs into an ungreased 6" round non-stick baking dish. Mix in butter, bell pepper, onion, ham, salt, and black pepper.

2 Place dish into air fryer basket. Adjust the temperature to 320°F and set the timer for 15 minutes. The eggs will be fully cooked and firm in the middle when done.

3 Slice in half and serve warm on two medium plates.

PER SERVING

CALORIES: 201	FAT: 14g
PROTEIN: 13g	SODIUM: 650mg
FIBER: 1g	CARBOHYDRATES: 3g
NET CARBOHYDRATES: 2g	SUGAR: 1g

Cinnamon Rolls

Don't be intimidated by the mozzarella—the cinnamon flavor will take over the mild taste of the cheese. If you enjoy a glaze, you can mix 1 tablespoon confectioners' erythritol with 3 tablespoons unsweetened almond milk or heavy whipping cream and drizzle it over the rolls when they have cooled.

- **Pantry Staples: Vanilla extract**
- **Hands-On Time: 10 minutes**
- **Cook Time: 20 minutes**

Yields 12 rolls

2½ cups shredded mozzarella cheese

2 ounces cream cheese, softened

1 cup blanched finely ground almond flour

½ teaspoon vanilla extract

½ cup confectioners' erythritol

1 tablespoon ground cinnamon

1 In a large microwave-safe bowl, combine mozzarella cheese, cream cheese, and flour. Microwave the mixture on high 90 seconds until cheese is melted.

2 Add vanilla extract and erythritol, and mix 2 minutes until a dough forms.

3 Once the dough is cool enough to work with your hands, about 2 minutes, spread it out into a 12″ × 4″ rectangle on ungreased parchment paper. Evenly sprinkle dough with cinnamon.

4 Starting at the long side of the dough, roll lengthwise to form a log. Slice the log into twelve even pieces.

5 Divide rolls between two ungreased 6″ round nonstick baking dishes. Place one dish into air fryer basket. Adjust the temperature to 375°F and set the timer for 10 minutes.

6 Cinnamon rolls will be done when golden around the edges and mostly firm. Repeat with second dish. Allow rolls to cool in dishes 10 minutes before serving.

PER SERVING (1 ROLL)

CALORIES: 145	**FAT:** 10g
PROTEIN: 8g	**SODIUM:** 177mg
FIBER: 1g	**CARBOHYDRATES:** 10g
NET CARBOHYDRATES: 3g	**SUGAR:** 1g
SUGAR ALCOHOL: 6g	

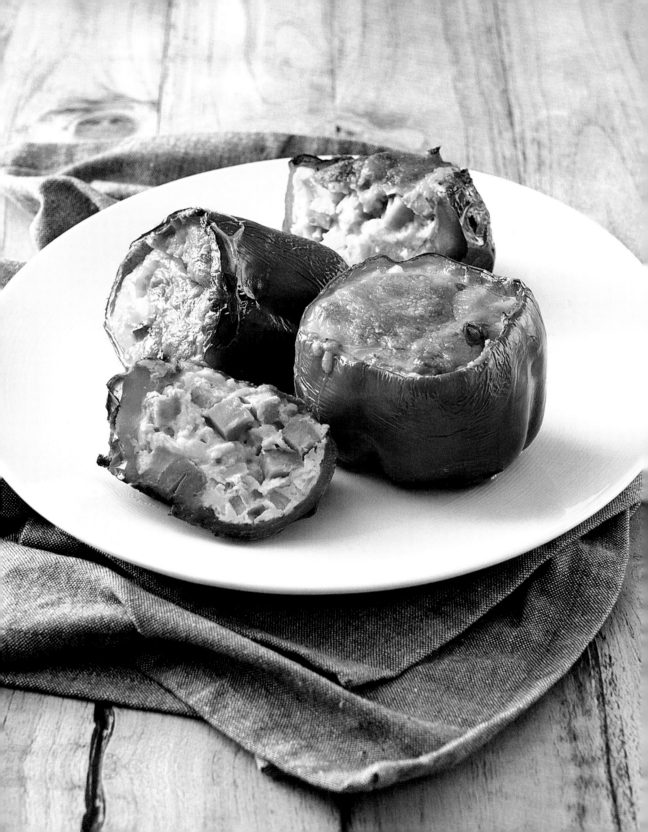

Cheesy Bell Pepper Eggs

This breakfast comes together quickly but isn't short on flavor. The eggs soak up the juices of the peppers, making for a delicious and fresh-tasting meal. Feel free to get creative and use your choice of cooked meat, such as crumbled sugar-free bacon.

- **Pantry Staples: Salt, coconut oil**
- **Hands-On Time: 10 minutes**
- **Cook Time: 15 minutes**

Serves 4

4 medium green bell peppers, tops removed, seeded

1 tablespoon coconut oil

3 ounces chopped cooked no-sugar-added ham

¼ cup peeled and chopped white onion

4 large eggs

½ teaspoon salt

1 cup shredded mild Cheddar cheese

1 Place peppers upright into ungreased air fryer basket. Drizzle each pepper with coconut oil. Divide ham and onion evenly among peppers.

2 In a medium bowl, whisk eggs, then sprinkle with salt. Pour mixture evenly into each pepper. Top each with ¼ cup Cheddar.

3 Adjust the temperature to 320°F and set the timer for 15 minutes. Peppers will be tender and eggs will be firm when done.

4 Serve warm on four medium plates.

PER SERVING

CALORIES: 281	FAT: 18g
PROTEIN: 18g	SODIUM: 767mg
FIBER: 2g	CARBOHYDRATES: 8g
NET CARBOHYDRATES: 6g	SUGAR: 4g

Egg White Cups

This recipe is perfect for when you're in the mood for something light. Egg whites take on the flavor of whatever you mix with them. Feel free to make these cups your own by adding mushrooms, ham, or a favorite seasoning blend.

- Pantry Staples: Salt
- Hands-On Time: 10 minutes
- Cook Time: 15 minutes

Serves 4

2 cups 100% liquid egg whites

3 tablespoons salted butter, melted

¼ teaspoon salt

¼ teaspoon onion powder

½ medium Roma tomato, cored and diced

½ cup chopped fresh spinach leaves

1 In a large bowl, whisk egg whites with butter, salt, and onion powder. Stir in tomato and spinach, then pour evenly into four 4" ramekins greased with cooking spray.

2 Place ramekins into air fryer basket. Adjust the temperature to 300°F and set the timer for 15 minutes. Eggs will be fully cooked and firm in the center when done. Serve warm.

PER SERVING

CALORIES: 146

PROTEIN: 14g

FIBER: 0g

NET CARBOHYDRATES: 1g

FAT: 8g

SODIUM: 416mg

CARBOHYDRATES: 1g

SUGAR: 0g

HIGH-PROTEIN MEALS

Just because keto is a high-fat diet doesn't mean you have to eat *only* high-fat foods. Protein is the first macro you should be sure to hit each day, so meals like these egg cups can be really handy when you feel hungry but are also watching your calories.

Spinach Omelet

Leafy green vegetables like spinach are a great part of a low-carb diet, as they are full of vitamins and fiber. This recipe is delicious and cheesy, and it will keep you going all morning.

- **Pantry Staples: Salt**
- **Hands-On Time: 5 minutes**
- **Cook Time: 12 minutes**

Serves 2

4 large eggs
1½ cups chopped fresh spinach leaves
2 tablespoons peeled and chopped yellow onion
2 tablespoons salted butter, melted
½ cup shredded mild Cheddar cheese
¼ teaspoon salt

1 In an ungreased 6" round nonstick baking dish, whisk eggs. Stir in spinach, onion, butter, Cheddar, and salt.

2 Place dish into air fryer basket. Adjust the temperature to 320°F and set the timer for 12 minutes. Omelet will be done when browned on the top and firm in the middle.

3 Slice in half and serve warm on two medium plates.

PER SERVING

CALORIES: 368	FAT: 28g
PROTEIN: 20g	SODIUM: 722mg
FIBER: 1g	CARBOHYDRATES: 3g
NET CARBOHYDRATES: 2g	SUGAR: 1g

Cheddar Soufflés

If you've ever been intimidated by soufflés, this recipe is for you. In less than 30 minutes you can enjoy this delicious breakfast. The light, cheesy taste pairs well with a couple of slices of sugar-free bacon or some fresh strawberries.

- **Pantry Staples: None**
- **Hands-On Time: 15 minutes**
- **Cook Time: 12 minutes**

Serves 4

3 large eggs, whites and
    yolks separated
¼ teaspoon cream of tartar
½ cup shredded sharp
    Cheddar cheese
3 ounces cream cheese,
    softened

1 In a large bowl, beat egg whites together with cream of tartar until soft peaks form, about 2 minutes.

2 In a separate medium bowl, beat egg yolks, Cheddar, and cream cheese together until frothy, about 1 minute. Add egg yolk mixture to whites, gently folding until combined.

3 Pour mixture evenly into four 4" ramekins greased with cooking spray. Place ramekins into air fryer basket. Adjust the temperature to 350°F and set the timer for 12 minutes. Eggs will be browned on the top and firm in the center when done. Serve warm.

PER SERVING

CALORIES: 183	**FAT:** 14g
PROTEIN: 9g	**SODIUM:** 221mg
FIBER: 0g	**CARBOHYDRATES:** 1g
NET CARBOHYDRATES: 1g	**SUGAR:** 1g

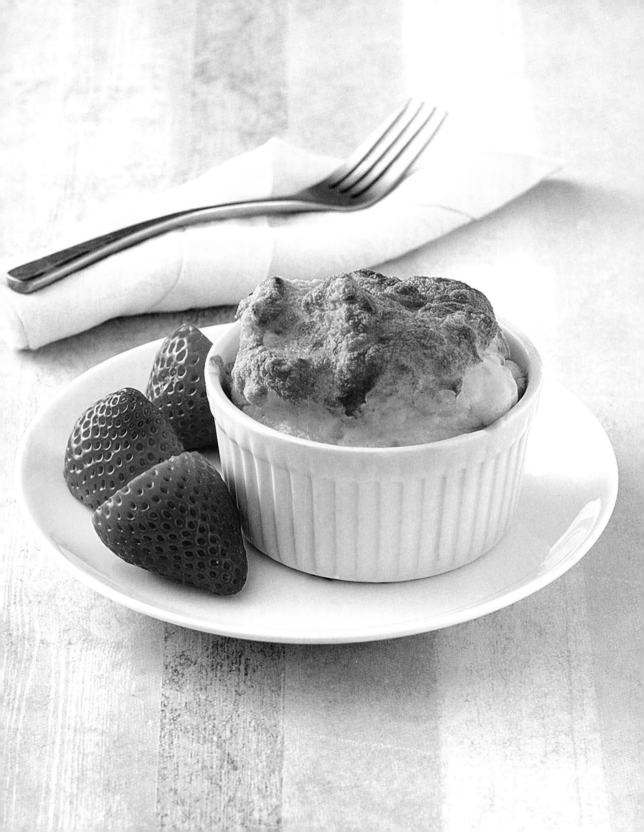

Bacon and Cheese Quiche

This meal gets back to basics with classic breakfast favorites: bacon and eggs. Every bite is so full of fluffy eggs, melted cheese, and crispy bacon that it will make you wish you'd doubled the recipe. But don't worry; they cook in less than 15 minutes, so you can quickly whip up another batch any time!

- **Pantry Staples: Salt**
- **Hands-On Time: 5 minutes**
- **Cook Time: 12 minutes**

Serves 2

3 large eggs

2 tablespoons heavy whipping cream

¼ teaspoon salt

4 slices cooked sugar-free bacon, crumbled

½ cup shredded mild Cheddar cheese

1 In a large bowl, whisk eggs, cream, and salt together until combined. Mix in bacon and Cheddar.

2 Pour mixture evenly into two ungreased 4" ramekins. Place into air fryer basket. Adjust the temperature to 320°F and set the timer for 12 minutes. Quiche will be fluffy and set in the middle when done.

3 Let quiche cool in ramekins 5 minutes. Serve warm.

PER SERVING

CALORIES: 380	FAT: 28g
PROTEIN: 24g	SODIUM: 971mg
FIBER: 0g	CARBOHYDRATES: 2g
NET CARBOHYDRATES: 2g	SUGAR: 1g

Breakfast Meatballs

These meatballs are perfect for breakfast on the go. You can easily double the recipe and keep them covered in the refrigerator for up to 1 week. Swap out the pork for turkey sausage if you prefer.

- **Pantry Staples: Salt, ground black pepper**
- **Hands-On Time: 10 minutes**
- **Cook Time: 15 minutes**

Yields 18 meatballs

1 pound ground pork
  breakfast sausage
½ teaspoon salt
¼ teaspoon ground black
  pepper
½ cup shredded sharp
  Cheddar cheese
1 ounce cream cheese,
  softened
1 large egg, whisked

1 Combine all ingredients in a large bowl. Form mixture into eighteen 1" meatballs.

2 Place meatballs into ungreased air fryer basket. Adjust the temperature to 400°F and set the timer for 15 minutes, shaking basket three times during cooking. Meatballs will be browned on the outside and have an internal temperature of at least 145°F when completely cooked. Serve warm.

PER SERVING (3 MEATBALLS)

CALORIES: 288

PROTEIN: 11g

FIBER: 0g

NET CARBOHYDRATES: 1g

FAT: 24g

SODIUM: 742mg

CARBOHYDRATES: 1g

SUGAR: 1g

Bunless Breakfast Turkey Burgers

This light breakfast will get you up and going without weighing you down. The juicy turkey patty gets a nice brown crust that seals in its flavors. Feel free to top with a fried egg or a drizzle of sriracha for a little heat.

- **Pantry Staples: Salt, ground black pepper**
- **Hands-On Time: 5 minutes**
- **Cook Time: 15 minutes**

Serves 4

1 pound ground turkey breakfast sausage
½ teaspoon salt
¼ teaspoon ground black pepper
¼ cup seeded and chopped green bell pepper
2 tablespoons mayonnaise
1 medium avocado, peeled, pitted, and sliced

1 In a large bowl, mix sausage with salt, black pepper, bell pepper, and mayonnaise. Form meat into four patties.

2 Place patties into ungreased air fryer basket. Adjust the temperature to 370°F and set the timer for 15 minutes, turning patties halfway through cooking. Burgers will be done when dark brown and they have an internal temperature of at least 165°F.

3 Serve burgers topped with avocado slices on four medium plates.

PER SERVING

CALORIES: 276	FAT: 17g
PROTEIN: 22g	SODIUM: 917mg
FIBER: 3g	CARBOHYDRATES: 4g
NET CARBOHYDRATES: 1g	SUGAR: 0g

Sausage-Crusted Egg Cups

Who doesn't love sausage and eggs for breakfast? This is a great recipe for a group that wants different add-ins. Everyone gets their own and can add their favorite chopped vegetables and seasonings. Try dipping in salsa and sour cream!

- **Pantry Staples: Salt, ground black pepper**
- **Hands-On Time: 10 minutes**
- **Cook Time: 15 minutes**

Serves 6

12 ounces ground pork breakfast sausage

6 large eggs

½ teaspoon salt

¼ teaspoon ground black pepper

½ teaspoon crushed red pepper flakes

1 Place sausage in six 4″ ramekins (about 2 ounces per ramekin) greased with cooking oil. Press sausage down to cover bottom and about ½″ up the sides of ramekins. Crack one egg into each ramekin and sprinkle evenly with salt, black pepper, and red pepper flakes.

2 Place ramekins into air fryer basket. Adjust the temperature to 350°F and set the timer for 15 minutes. Egg cups will be done when sausage is fully cooked to at least 145°F and the egg is firm. Serve warm.

PER SERVING

CALORIES: 267

PROTEIN: 14g

FIBER: 0g

NET CARBOHYDRATES: 1g

FAT: 21g

SODIUM: 679mg

CARBOHYDRATES: 1g

SUGAR: 0g

Mini Bagels

Bagels are a classic quick and easy breakfast, but the carb count of the traditional bagel is too high for a keto diet. These Mini Bagels will give you what you've been missing—without compromising your keto goals. Serve with cream cheese and everything bagel seasoning to round out the flavor!

- **Pantry Staples: Baking powder**
- **Hands-On Time: 5 minutes**
- **Cook Time: 10 minutes**

Yields 6 mini bagels

2 cups blanched finely ground almond flour

2 cups shredded mozzarella cheese

3 tablespoons salted butter, divided

1½ teaspoons baking powder

1 teaspoon apple cider vinegar

2 large eggs, divided

1 In a large microwave-safe bowl, combine flour, mozzarella, and 1 tablespoon butter. Microwave on high 90 seconds, then form into a soft ball of dough.

2 Add baking powder, vinegar, and 1 egg to dough, stirring until fully combined.

3 Once dough is cool enough to work with your hands, about 2 minutes, divide evenly into six balls. Poke a hole in each ball of dough with your finger and gently stretch each ball out to be 2" in diameter.

4 In a small microwave-safe bowl, melt remaining butter in microwave on high 30 seconds, then let cool 1 minute. Whisk with remaining egg, then brush mixture over each bagel.

5 Line air fryer basket with parchment paper and place bagels onto ungreased parchment, working in batches if needed.

6 Adjust the temperature to 350°F and set the timer for 10 minutes. Halfway through, use tongs to flip bagels for even cooking.

7 Allow bagels to set and cool completely, about 15 minutes, before serving. Store leftovers in a sealed bag in the refrigerator up to 4 days.

PER SERVING (1 MINI BAGEL)

CALORIES: 415	**FAT:** 33g
PROTEIN: 19g	**SODIUM:** 447mg
FIBER: 4g	**CARBOHYDRATES:** 10g
NET CARBOHYDRATES: 6g	**SUGAR:** 2g

Jalapeño and Bacon Breakfast Pizza

If you love jalapeño poppers, you'll be a huge fan of this jalapeño- and bacon-covered breakfast. The cheese and egg make a creamy crust that pairs perfectly with spicy peppers for a mouthwatering meal. It's an indulgent recipe that still keeps you on track.

- **Pantry Staples:** Salt
- **Hands-On Time:** 5 minutes
- **Cook Time:** 10 minutes

Serves 2

1 cup shredded mozzarella cheese

1 ounce cream cheese, broken into small pieces

4 slices cooked sugar-free bacon, chopped

¼ cup chopped pickled jalapeños

1 large egg, whisked

¼ teaspoon salt

1 Place mozzarella in a single layer on the bottom of an ungreased 6" round nonstick baking dish. Scatter cream cheese pieces, bacon, and jalapeños over mozzarella, then pour egg evenly around baking dish.

2 Sprinkle with salt and place into air fryer basket. Adjust the temperature to 330°F and set the timer for 10 minutes. When cheese is brown and egg is set, pizza will be done.

3 Let cool on a large plate 5 minutes before serving.

PER SERVING

CALORIES: 361	**FAT:** 24g
PROTEIN: 26g	**SODIUM:** 1,324mg
FIBER: 0g	**CARBOHYDRATES:** 5g
NET CARBOHYDRATES: 5g	**SUGAR:** 2g

Pizza Eggs

Savory herbs and filling protein make this a great brunch option. To make this meal even more filling, add your favorite chopped vegetables, such as mushrooms or spinach, or 2 tablespoons low-carb marinara to make it taste even more like pizza.

- **Pantry Staples: Salt, garlic powder**
- **Hands-On Time: 5 minutes**
- **Cook Time: 10 minutes**

Serves 2

1 cup shredded mozzarella cheese
7 slices pepperoni, chopped
1 large egg, whisked
¼ teaspoon dried oregano
¼ teaspoon dried parsley
¼ teaspoon garlic powder
¼ teaspoon salt

1 Place mozzarella in a single layer on the bottom of an ungreased 6″ round nonstick baking dish. Scatter pepperoni over cheese, then pour egg evenly around baking dish.

2 Sprinkle with remaining ingredients and place into air fryer basket. Adjust the temperature to 330°F and set the timer for 10 minutes. When cheese is brown and egg is set, dish will be done.

3 Let cool in dish 5 minutes before serving.

PER SERVING

CALORIES: 241	FAT: 15g
PROTEIN: 19g	SODIUM: 834mg
FIBER: 0g	CARBOHYDRATES: 4g
NET CARBOHYDRATES: 4g	SUGAR: 1g

Cheesy Cauliflower "Hash Browns"

Cauliflower has a great texture and neutral flavor that allows it to replicate your favorite potato dishes. This recipe uses ground cheese crisps, which can often be found near the deli section of your grocery store. Brands like Whisps and Parm Crisps are excellent options that contain only cheese and no flour fillers.

- **Pantry Staples: Salt**
- **Hands-On Time: 30 minutes**
- **Cook Time: 24 minutes**

Yields 6 hash browns

2 ounces 100% cheese crisps
1 (12-ounce) steamer bag cauliflower, cooked according to package instructions
1 large egg
½ cup shredded sharp Cheddar cheese
½ teaspoon salt

STEAMER BAGS

This recipe uses a steamer bag of cauliflower to cut down on prep time. Feel free to swap for fresh cauliflower cooked using your preferred method. As long as it's tender and excess water is removed before placing into the food processor, it will work the same.

1 Let cooked cauliflower cool 10 minutes.

2 Place cheese crisps into food processor and pulse on low 30 seconds until crisps are finely ground.

3 Using a kitchen towel, wring out excess moisture from cauliflower and place into food processor.

4 Add egg to food processor and sprinkle with Cheddar and salt. Pulse five times until mixture is mostly smooth.

5 Cut two pieces of parchment to fit air fryer basket. Separate mixture into six even scoops and place three on each piece of ungreased parchment, keeping at least 2" of space between each scoop. Press each into a hash brown shape, about ¼" thick.

6 Place one batch on parchment into air fryer basket. Adjust the temperature to 375°F and set the timer for 12 minutes, turning hash browns halfway through cooking. Hash browns will be golden brown when done. Repeat with second batch.

7 Allow 5 minutes to cool. Serve warm.

PER SERVING (1 HASH BROWN)

CALORIES: 120
PROTEIN: 8g
FIBER: 1g
NET CARBOHYDRATES: 2g
FAT: 8g
SODIUM: 390mg
CARBOHYDRATES: 3g
SUGAR: 1g

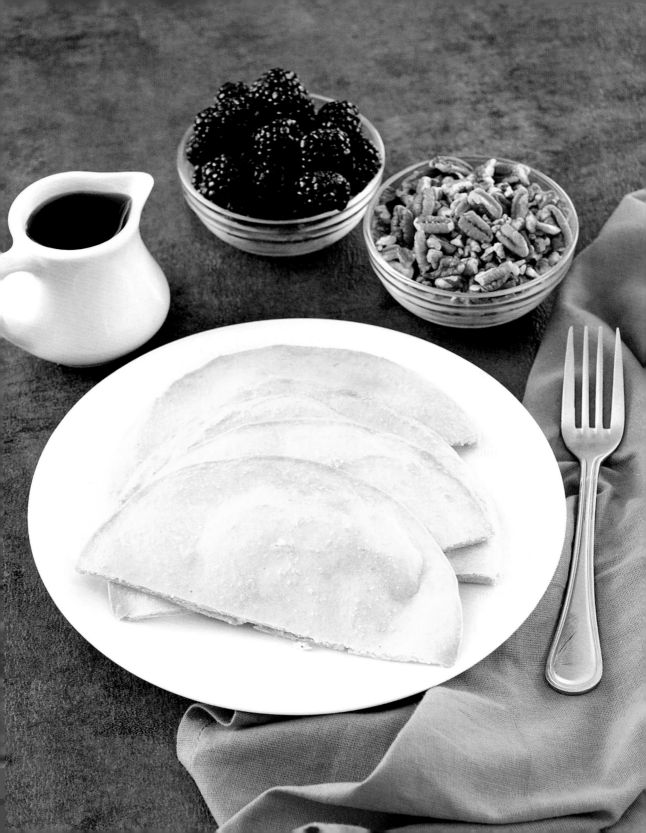

Pancake for Two

This recipe is an easy spin on a breakfast classic. You get all the fluffy pancake goodness that you love in minutes (and fewer carbs!). Use this recipe as a base and get creative with your favorite flavor extracts and add-ins. Chopped nuts, blackberries, and low-carb maple syrup make great toppings and will easily take this recipe to the next level.

- **Pantry Staples: Vanilla extract**
- **Hands-On Time: 5 minutes**
- **Cook Time: 30 minutes**

Serves 2

1 cup blanched finely ground almond flour

2 tablespoons granular erythritol

1 tablespoon salted butter, melted

1 large egg

⅓ cup unsweetened almond milk

½ teaspoon vanilla extract

1 In a large bowl, mix all ingredients together, then pour half the batter into an ungreased 6" round nonstick baking dish.

2 Place dish into air fryer basket. Adjust the temperature to 320°F and set the timer for 15 minutes. The pancake will be golden brown on top and firm, and a toothpick inserted in the center will come out clean when done. Repeat with remaining batter.

3 Slice in half in dish and serve warm.

PER SERVING

CALORIES: 434	FAT: 38g
PROTEIN: 15g	SODIUM: 111mg
FIBER: 6g	CARBOHYDRATES: 23g
NET CARBOHYDRATES: 5g	SUGAR: 2g
SUGAR ALCOHOL: 12g	

LOW-CARB MAPLE SYRUPS

Just because a maple syrup is low in sugar or sugar-free doesn't mean it's always the best option. Some syrups may use high-glycemic sweeteners that can spike blood sugar levels. Look for options that use sweeteners such as monk fruit or erythritol, like ChocZero and Lakanto.

Scotch Eggs

A batch of hard-boiled eggs can be great for meal prep, but this recipe takes things to the next level. The eggs are wrapped in flavorful sausage for a more complete meal. The extra fat from the sausage will keep you full and give you the energy needed to get through the day.

- **Pantry Staples: Salt, ground black pepper**
- **Hands-On Time: 10 minutes**
- **Cook Time: 12 minutes**

Yields 8 eggs

1 large egg, whisked

1 pound ground pork breakfast sausage

½ cup blanched finely ground almond flour

½ teaspoon salt

¼ teaspoon ground black pepper

8 large hard-boiled eggs, shells removed

1 In a large bowl, mix raw egg with sausage, flour, salt, and pepper.

2 Form ¼ cup of the mixture around 1 hard-boiled egg, completely covering the egg. Repeat with remaining mixture and hard-boiled eggs.

3 Place eggs into ungreased air fryer basket. Adjust the temperature to 400°F and set the timer for 12 minutes, turning halfway through cooking. Eggs will be done when browned. Let eggs cool 5 minutes before serving.

PER SERVING (1 EGG)

CALORIES: 325	**FAT:** 25g
PROTEIN: 17g	**SODIUM:** 630mg
FIBER: 1g	**CARBOHYDRATES:** 2g
NET CARBOHYDRATES: 1g	**SUGAR:** 1g

Cinnamon Granola

If you've been missing that cereal crunch while on a keto diet, this recipe is for you! You can enjoy it with unsweetened almond milk or sprinkled over low-carb yogurt. Feel free to add your favorite nuts and seeds, or even low-carb chocolate chips.

- Pantry Staples: None
- Hands-On Time: 10 minutes
- Cook Time: 7 minutes

Yields 4 cups

2 cups shelled pecans, chopped

1 cup unsweetened coconut flakes

1 cup slivered almonds

2 tablespoons granular erythritol

1 teaspoon ground cinnamon

1. In a large bowl, mix all ingredients. Place mixture into an ungreased 6″ round nonstick baking dish.

2. Place dish into air fryer basket. Adjust the temperature to 320°F and set the timer for 7 minutes, stirring halfway through cooking.

3. Let cool in dish 10 minutes before serving. Store in airtight container at room temperature up to 5 days.

PER SERVING (⅔ CUP)

CALORIES: 445
PROTEIN: 8g
FIBER: 9g
NET CARBOHYDRATES: 4g
SUGAR ALCOHOL: 4g

FAT: 42g
SODIUM: 0mg
CARBOHYDRATES: 17g
SUGAR: 3g

LOW-CARB YOGURT

There's a growing number of low-carb yogurts on the market. Since yogurt is dairy, you're likely to see some natural sugar on the label—and that's okay. Just be sure to look for full-fat yogurts without added sugar.

Jalapeño Egg Cups

The savory goodness of a classic appetizer has finally come to the breakfast table! Spice up your morning with eggs that pack a serious punch. Be sure to make enough for second helpings—you'll be glad you did.

- **Pantry Staples: Salt, ground black pepper, garlic powder**
- **Hands-On Time: 10 minutes**
- **Cook Time: 14 minutes**

Serves 4

4 large eggs

½ teaspoon salt

¼ teaspoon ground black pepper

¼ cup chopped pickled jalapeños

2 ounces cream cheese, softened

¼ teaspoon garlic powder

½ cup shredded sharp Cheddar cheese

1 In a medium bowl, beat eggs together with salt and pepper, then pour evenly into four 4" ramekins greased with cooking spray.

2 In a separate large bowl, mix jalapeños, cream cheese, garlic powder, and Cheddar. Spoon ¼ of the mixture into the center of one ramekin. Repeat with remaining mixture and ramekins.

3 Place ramekins in air fryer basket. Adjust the temperature to 320°F and set the timer for 14 minutes. Eggs will be set when done. Serve warm.

PER SERVING

CALORIES: 177

PROTEIN: 11g

FIBER: 0g

NET CARBOHYDRATES: 1g

FAT: 13g

SODIUM: 591mg

CARBOHYDRATES: 1g

SUGAR: 1g

Appetizers and Snacks

Whether it's midday or game day, appetizers and snacks are a fun way to help tide you over between meals. Because of the comforting nature of these treats, however, it can be a bit tough to find satisfying snacks that are keto friendly. Luckily, the air fryer makes snacking easy *and* healthy. Plus, there are smart swaps for just about every carb-filled favorite.

From Bacon-Wrapped Jalapeño Poppers and Pepperoni Rolls to Three Cheese Dip and Avocado Fries, this chapter is full of mouthwatering, five-ingredient appetizers and snacks that will give your day a little something extra—without derailing your diet!

Broccoli and Carrot Bites

This recipe is the perfect snack because it's vegetable-based and low in calories while still being delicious and satisfying. It's a smart option to keep you on track.

- **Pantry Staples: Salt, ground black pepper**
- **Hands-On Time: 15 minutes**
- **Cook Time: 12 minutes**

Yields 20 bites

1 (10-ounce) steamer bag broccoli, cooked according to package instructions

½ cup shredded sharp Cheddar cheese

2 tablespoons peeled and grated carrot

½ cup blanched finely ground almond flour

1 large egg, whisked

¼ teaspoon salt

¼ teaspoon ground black pepper

1 Let cooked broccoli cool 5 minutes, then wring out excess moisture with a kitchen towel. In a large bowl, mix broccoli with Cheddar, carrot, flour, egg, salt, and pepper. Scoop 2 tablespoons of the mixture into a ball, then roll into a bite-sized piece. Repeat with remaining mixture to form twenty bites.

2 Cut a piece of parchment to fit into the bottom of air fryer basket. Place bites into a single layer on ungreased parchment. Adjust the temperature to 320°F and set the timer for 12 minutes, turning bites halfway through cooking. Bites will be golden brown when done. Serve warm.

PER SERVING (5 BITES)

CALORIES: 191	**FAT:** 13g
PROTEIN: 10g	**SODIUM:** 291mg
FIBER: 5g	**CARBOHYDRATES:** 9g
NET CARBOHYDRATES: 4g	**SUGAR:** 3g

IT'S KID FRIENDLY!

This recipe is a great way to get the kiddos to enjoy some vegetables! Ranch and low-carb ketchup are perfect choices for dipping and will make kids excited about eating vegetables.

Bacon-Wrapped Jalapeño Poppers

These poppers are the ultimate savory treat, crisped to perfection in the air fryer. With a blend of creamy, cheesy, and spicy flavors, they're ideal for your game day spread. They also reheat well, so feel free to double the recipe and store in the refrigerator up to 5 days.

- Pantry Staples: Garlic powder
- Hands-On Time: 10 minutes
- Cook Time: 12 minutes

Yields 12 poppers

3 ounces cream cheese, softened

⅓ cup shredded mild Cheddar cheese

¼ teaspoon garlic powder

6 jalapeños (approximately 4" long), tops removed, sliced in half lengthwise and seeded

12 slices sugar-free bacon

1 Place cream cheese, Cheddar, and garlic powder in a large microwave-safe bowl. Microwave 30 seconds on high, then stir. Spoon cheese mixture evenly into hollowed jalapeños.

2 Wrap 1 slice bacon around each jalapeño half, completely covering jalapeño, and secure with a toothpick. Place jalapeños into ungreased air fryer basket. Adjust the temperature to 400°F and set the timer for 12 minutes, turning jalapeños halfway through cooking. Bacon will be crispy when done. Serve warm.

PER SERVING (3 POPPERS)

CALORIES: 278	FAT: 21g
PROTEIN: 15g	SODIUM: 719mg
FIBER: 1g	CARBOHYDRATES: 3g
NET CARBOHYDRATES: 2g	SUGAR: 2g

Spicy Cheese-Stuffed Mushrooms

This appetizer is great on a budget and packs big flavor with just a few ingredients. The mushrooms get a crispy exterior while cooking that is complemented by the tender, cheesy stuffing. If you prefer things milder, swap the pepper jack cheese for Monterey jack cheese.

- **Pantry Staples: Salt, ground black pepper**
- **Hands-On Time: 10 minutes**
- **Cook Time: 8 minutes**

Yields 20 mushrooms

4 ounces cream cheese, softened

6 tablespoons shredded pepper jack cheese

2 tablespoons chopped pickled jalapeños

20 medium button mushrooms, stems removed

2 tablespoons olive oil

¼ teaspoon salt

⅛ teaspoon ground black pepper

1 In a large bowl, mix cream cheese, pepper jack, and jalapeños together.

2 Drizzle mushrooms with olive oil, then sprinkle with salt and pepper. Spoon 2 tablespoons cheese mixture into each mushroom and place in a single layer into ungreased air fryer basket. Adjust the temperature to 370°F and set the timer for 8 minutes, checking halfway through cooking to ensure even cooking, rearranging if some are darker than others. When they're golden and cheese is bubbling, mushrooms will be done. Serve warm.

PER SERVING (2 MUSHROOMS)

CALORIES: 87	**FAT:** 7g
PROTEIN: 3g	**SODIUM:** 144mg
FIBER: 0g	**CARBOHYDRATES:** 2g
NET CARBOHYDRATES: 2g	**SUGAR:** 1g

MILD VERSUS SPICY JALAPEÑOS

If you don't like spicy food, consider trying mild pickled jalapeños. These often have the seeds and membrane removed (which give the pepper most of its heat). They can be a good option if you want to enjoy the flavor without the heat.

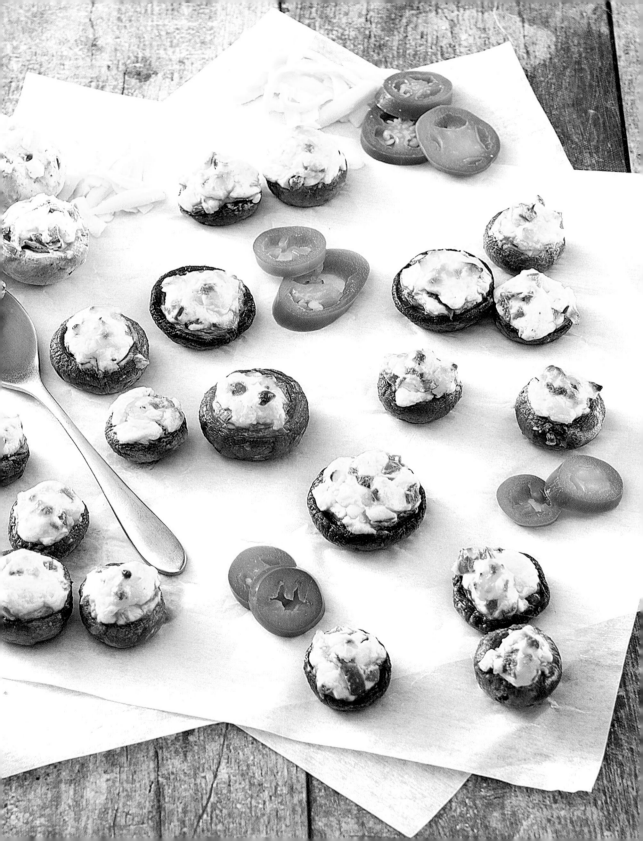

Pepperoni Chips

Classic potato chips, even the baked variety, can have as many as 23 grams of carbs per serving. Fortunately, you don't have to sacrifice that crispy, savory flavor when on a keto diet—just whip up a quick batch of these delicious, protein-rich Pepperoni Chips.

- Pantry Staples: None
- Hands-On Time: 5 minutes
- Cook Time: 8 minutes

Serves 2

14 slices pepperoni

MAKE IT MORE FILLING
You can turn these chips into a hearty snack by pairing with your favorite dip, or stacking them with cuts of Cheddar cheese!

Place pepperoni slices into ungreased air fryer basket. Adjust the temperature to 350°F and set the timer for 8 minutes. Pepperoni will be browned and crispy when done. Let cool 5 minutes before serving. Store in airtight container at room temperature up to 3 days.

PER SERVING

CALORIES: 69	FAT: 5g
PROTEIN: 3g	SODIUM: 246mg
FIBER: 0g	CARBOHYDRATES: 0g
NET CARBOHYDRATES: 0g	SUGAR: 0g

Bacon-Wrapped Onion Rings

These onion rings are easier to make than the traditional deep-fried version! The savory taste of the onion is paired with salty bacon to create a delicious side you'll want to make regularly.

- Pantry Staples: None
- Hands-On Time: 5 minutes
- Cook Time: 10 minutes

Serves 8

1 large white onion, peeled and cut into 16 (¼"-thick) slices
8 slices sugar-free bacon

1 Stack 2 slices onion and wrap with 1 slice bacon. Secure with a toothpick. Repeat with remaining onion slices and bacon.

2 Place onion rings into ungreased air fryer basket. Adjust the temperature to 350°F and set the timer for 10 minutes, turning rings halfway through cooking. Bacon will be crispy when done. Serve warm.

PER SERVING

CALORIES: 84	FAT: 4g
PROTEIN: 5g	SODIUM: 197mg
FIBER: 2g	CARBOHYDRATES: 8g
NET CARBOHYDRATES: 6g	SUGAR: 3g

Three Cheese Dip

Whether you prefer vegetables or pork rinds and cheese cr.
ultracreamy recipe is sure to be a winner. Add your own flair
chicken, chopped scallions, or hot sauce.

- Pantry Staples: None
- Hands-On Time: 5 minutes
- Cook Time: 12 minutes

Serves 8 (Yields 1 cup)

8 ounces cream cheese, softened
½ cup mayonnaise
¼ cup sour cream
½ cup shredded sharp
   Cheddar cheese
¼ cup shredded Monterey
   jack cheese

1 In a large bowl, con
   mixture into an ung
   baking dish and pla

2 Adjust the temperature to 375°F and set the
   timer for 12 minutes. Dip will be browned on
   top and bubbling when done. Serve warm.

PER SERVING (2 TABLESPOONS)

CALORIES: 245	FAT: 23g
PROTEIN: 5g	SODIUM: 260mg
FIBER: 0g	CARBOHYDRATES: 2g
NET CARBOHYDRATES: 2g	SUGAR: 1g

Buffalo Chicken Dip

Just because you don't eat traditional chips on a keto diet doesn't mean your days of
delicious dips are over. This dip is tasty paired with 100% cheese crisps such as Parm
Crisps, or tossed into your morning omelet.

- Pantry Staples: None
- Hands-On Time: 10 minutes
- Cook Time: 12 minutes

Serves 8 (Yields 4 cups)

8 ounces cream cheese,
   softened
2 cups chopped cooked
   chicken thighs
½ cup buffalo sauce
1 cup shredded mild Cheddar
   cheese, divided

1 In a large bowl, combine cream cheese,
   chicken, buffalo sauce, and ½ cup Cheddar.
   Scoop dip into an ungreased 4-cup nonstick
   baking dish and top with remaining Cheddar.

2 Place dish into air fryer basket. Adjust the
   temperature to 375°F and set the timer for
   12 minutes. Dip will be browned on top and
   bubbling when done. Serve warm.

PER SERVING (½ CUP)

CALORIES: 222	FAT: 15g
PROTEIN: 14g	SODIUM: 680mg
FIBER: 0g	CARBOHYDRATES: 1g
NET CARBOHYDRATES: 1g	SUGAR: 1g

...roni Rolls

...y, cheesy rolls are a kid-friendly keto snack for any time of day. Who wouldn't ...extra-cheesy bite of classic pizza flavors? Be sure to serve them with a low-carb ...nara sauce on the side for dipping!

- **Pantry Staples: None**
- **Hands-On Time: 5 minutes**
- **Cook Time: 8 minutes**

Yields 12 rolls

2½ cups shredded mozzarella cheese

2 ounces cream cheese, softened

1 cup blanched finely ground almond flour

48 slices pepperoni

2 teaspoons Italian seasoning

1. In a large microwave-safe bowl, combine mozzarella, cream cheese, and flour. Microwave on high 90 seconds until cheese is melted.

2. Using a wooden spoon, mix melted mixture 2 minutes until a dough forms.

3. Once dough is cool enough to work with your hands, about 2 minutes, spread it out into a 12" × 4" rectangle on ungreased parchment paper. Line dough with pepperoni, divided into four even rows. Sprinkle Italian seasoning evenly over pepperoni.

4. Starting at the long end of the dough, roll up until a log is formed. Slice the log into twelve even pieces.

5. Place pizza rolls in an ungreased 6" nonstick baking dish. Adjust the temperature to 375°F and set the timer for 8 minutes. Rolls will be golden and firm when done. Allow cooked rolls to cool 10 minutes before serving.

PER SERVING (2 ROLLS)

CALORIES: 366	**FAT:** 27g
PROTEIN: 20g	**SODIUM:** 637mg
FIBER: 2g	**CARBOHYDRATES:** 7g
NET CARBOHYDRATES: 5g	**SUGAR:** 2g

Cauliflower Buns

There is no end to cauliflower's versatility! These buns give you a breadlike consistency without the carbs (or the density of many low-carb bread replacements). They're also full of nutrients and will make the perfect companion to your next burger!

- Pantry Staples: Salt
- Hands-On Time: 15 minutes
- Cook Time: 12 minutes

Yields 8 buns

1 (12-ounce) steamer bag cauliflower, cooked according to package instructions
½ cup shredded mozzarella cheese
¼ cup shredded mild Cheddar cheese
¼ cup blanched finely ground almond flour
1 large egg
½ teaspoon salt

EXCESS WATER

Cauliflower carries a lot more moisture than most vegetables, so it's important to squeeze out excess water before cooking. These buns will only get solid and crispy when the cauliflower is thoroughly wrung out using a kitchen towel or cheesecloth.

1 Let cooked cauliflower cool about 10 minutes. Use a kitchen towel to wring out excess moisture, then place cauliflower in a food processor.

2 Add mozzarella, Cheddar, flour, egg, and salt to the food processor and pulse twenty times until mixture is combined. It will resemble a soft, wet dough.

3 Divide mixture into eight piles. Wet your hands with water to prevent sticking, then press each pile into a flat bun shape, about ½" thick.

4 Cut a sheet of parchment to fit air fryer basket. Working in batches if needed, place the formed dough onto ungreased parchment in air fryer basket. Adjust the temperature to 350°F and set the timer for 12 minutes, turning buns halfway through cooking.

5 Let buns cool 10 minutes before serving. Serve warm.

PER SERVING (1 BUN)

CALORIES: 75	FAT: 5g
PROTEIN: 5g	SODIUM: 235mg
FIBER: 1g	CARBOHYDRATES: 3g
NET CARBOHYDRATES: 2g	SUGAR: 1g

Mini Greek Meatballs

This recipe is great for potlucks and get-togethers as the perfect way to show off how delicious keto foods can be. It's all the best turkey burger toppings rolled into one little bite. Serve on toothpicks alongside cucumbers and cherry tomatoes with tzatziki sauce for dipping.

- **Pantry Staples: Salt, ground black pepper**
- **Hands-On Time: 10 minutes**
- **Cook Time: 10 minutes**

Yields 36 meatballs

1 cup fresh spinach leaves
¼ cup peeled and diced red onion
½ cup crumbled feta cheese
1 pound 85/15 ground turkey
½ teaspoon salt
½ teaspoon ground cumin
¼ teaspoon ground black pepper

MEAL PREP MEATBALLS

These meatballs reheat great in the microwave, so make a batch (or two!) to refrigerate in a sealed container for up to 5 days. Place a few meatballs on top of a cup of buttery cooked cauliflower rice for a filling lunch.

1 Place spinach, onion, and feta in a food processor, and pulse ten times until spinach is chopped. Scoop into a large bowl.

2 Add turkey to bowl and sprinkle with salt, cumin, and pepper. Mix until fully combined. Roll mixture into thirty-six meatballs (about 1 tablespoon each).

3 Place meatballs into ungreased air fryer basket, working in batches if needed. Adjust the temperature to 350°F and set the timer for 10 minutes, shaking basket twice during cooking. Meatballs will be browned and have an internal temperature of at least 165°F when done. Serve warm.

PER SERVING (4 MEATBALLS)

CALORIES: 115
PROTEIN: 10g
FIBER: 0g
NET CARBOHYDRATES: 1g

FAT: 7g
SODIUM: 235mg
CARBOHYDRATES: 1g
SUGAR: 1g

Sweet and Spicy Beef Jerky

Most commercial beef jerky is loaded with sugar, which makes it softer and improves flavor. With your air fryer, you can replicate that irresistible flavor and texture—without the carbs.

- **Pantry Staples: Ground black pepper**
- **Hands-On Time: 2 hours**
- **Cook Time: 4 hours**

Serves 6

1 pound eye of round beef, fat trimmed, sliced into ¼"-thick strips
¼ cup soy sauce
2 tablespoons sriracha hot chili sauce
½ teaspoon ground black pepper
2 tablespoons granular brown erythritol

1 Place beef in a large sealable bowl or bag. Pour soy sauce and sriracha into bowl or bag, then sprinkle in pepper and erythritol. Shake or stir to combine ingredients and coat steak. Cover and place in refrigerator to marinate at least 2 hours up to overnight.

2 Once marinated, remove strips from marinade and pat dry. Place into ungreased air fryer basket in a single layer, working in batches if needed. Adjust the temperature to 180°F and set the timer for 4 hours. Jerky will be chewy and dark brown when done. Store in airtight container in a cool, dry place up to 2 weeks.

PER SERVING

CALORIES: 99	FAT: 2g
PROTEIN: 18g	SODIUM: 381mg
FIBER: 0g	CARBOHYDRATES: 3g
NET CARBOHYDRATES: 1g	SUGAR: 1g
SUGAR ALCOHOL: 2g	

Crispy Deviled Eggs

This crispy spin on a classic appetizer will be the talk of your next party. If you like things spicy, add 2 teaspoons hot sauce to the egg yolks before spooning into the whites for a little burst of heat.

- **Pantry Staples: Salt, ground black pepper**
- **Hands-On Time: 10 minutes**
- **Cook Time: 25 minutes**

Yields 12 eggs

7 large eggs, divided
1 ounce plain pork rinds, finely crushed
2 tablespoons mayonnaise
¼ teaspoon salt
¼ teaspoon ground black pepper

HARD-BOILED EGGS IN THE AIR FRYER

Did you know that you don't have to turn on the stove to hard-boil your eggs? Just set the whole eggs in your air fryer basket at 220°F for 20 minutes. No water necessary!

1   Place 6 whole eggs into ungreased air fryer basket. Adjust the temperature to 220°F and set the timer for 20 minutes. When done, place eggs into a bowl of ice water to cool 5 minutes.

2   Peel cool eggs, then cut in half lengthwise. Remove yolks and place aside in a medium bowl.

3   In a separate small bowl, whisk remaining raw egg. Place pork rinds in a separate medium bowl. Dip each egg white into whisked egg, then gently coat with pork rinds. Spritz with cooking spray and place into ungreased air fryer basket. Adjust the temperature to 400°F and set the timer for 5 minutes, turning eggs halfway through cooking. Eggs will be golden when done.

4   Mash yolks in bowl with mayonnaise until smooth. Sprinkle with salt and pepper and mix.

5   Spoon 2 tablespoons yolk mixture into each fried egg white. Serve warm.

PER SERVING (2 EGGS)

CALORIES: 141	FAT: 10g
PROTEIN: 10g	SODIUM: 286mg
FIBER: 0g	CARBOHYDRATES: 1g
NET CARBOHYDRATES: 1g	SUGAR: 0g

Bacon-Wrapped Cabbage Bites

Sometimes getting your vegetables in requires a little creativity. These bites are excellent as an appetizer or main dish. The bacon flavor cooks into the cabbage, which gets crisp on the edges as it roasts and caramelizes. Feel free to add your own spices, such as Cajun seasoning, for a twist.

- **Pantry Staples: Salt, garlic powder, coconut oil**
- **Hands-On Time: 10 minutes**
- **Cook Time: 12 minutes**

Serves 6

3 tablespoons sriracha hot chili sauce, divided

1 medium head cabbage, cored and cut into 12 bite-sized pieces

2 tablespoons coconut oil, melted

½ teaspoon salt

12 slices sugar-free bacon

½ cup mayonnaise

¼ teaspoon garlic powder

1 Evenly brush 2 tablespoons sriracha onto cabbage pieces. Drizzle evenly with coconut oil, then sprinkle with salt.

2 Wrap each cabbage piece with bacon and secure with a toothpick. Place into ungreased air fryer basket. Adjust the temperature to 375°F and set the timer for 12 minutes, turning cabbage halfway through cooking. Bacon will be cooked and crispy when done.

3 In a small bowl, whisk together mayonnaise, garlic powder, and remaining sriracha. Use as a dipping sauce for cabbage bites.

PER SERVING

CALORIES: 316	FAT: 26g
PROTEIN: 10g	SODIUM: 874mg
FIBER: 4g	CARBOHYDRATES: 11g
NET CARBOHYDRATES: 7g	SUGAR: 6g

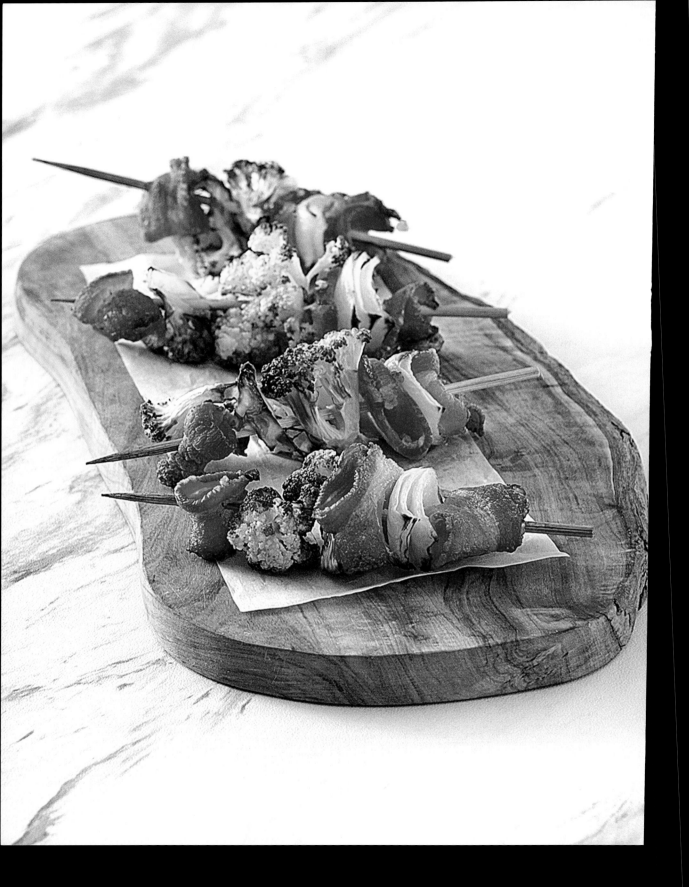

Bacon-y Cauliflower Skewers

This recipe can be prepped ahead of time in the morning to make dinnertime easier. The cauliflower gets golden brown and creates a delicious bite paired with the sweet onion. To reheat, adjust the temperature to 400°F and set the timer for 3 minutes.

- **Pantry Staples: Salt, garlic powder**
- **Hands-On Time: 10 minutes**
- **Cook Time: 12 minutes**

Serves 4

4 slices sugar-free bacon, cut into thirds

¼ medium yellow onion, peeled and cut into 1" pieces

4 ounces (about 8) cauliflower florets

1½ tablespoons olive oil

¼ teaspoon salt

¼ teaspoon garlic powder

1 Place 1 piece bacon and 2 pieces onion on a 6" skewer. Add a second piece bacon, and 2 cauliflower florets, followed by another piece of bacon onto skewer. Repeat with remaining ingredients and three additional skewers to make four total skewers.

2 Drizzle skewers with olive oil, then sprinkle with salt and garlic powder. Place skewers into ungreased air fryer basket. Adjust the temperature to 375°F and set the timer for 12 minutes, turning the skewers halfway through cooking. When done, vegetables will be tender and bacon will be crispy. Serve warm.

PER SERVING

CALORIES: 69	**FAT:** 5g
PROTEIN: 5g	**SODIUM:** 347mg
FIBER: 1g	**CARBOHYDRATES:** 2g
NET CARBOHYDRATES: 1g	**SUGAR:** 1g

Sausage-Stuffed Mushrooms

Try these tasty, healthy mushrooms to keep your energy up and appetite down.

- **Pantry Staples: Salt, garlic powder**
- **Hands-On Time: 10 minutes**
- **Cook Time: 20 minutes**

Serves 6

½ pound ground pork sausage

¼ teaspoon salt

¼ teaspoon garlic powder

2 medium scallions, trimmed and chopped

½ ounce plain pork rinds, finely crushed

1 pound cremini mushrooms, stems removed

1 In a large bowl, mix sausage, salt, garlic powder, scallions, and pork rinds. Scoop 1 tablespoon mixture into center of each mushroom cap.

2 Place mushrooms into ungreased air fryer basket. Adjust the temperature to 375°F and set the timer for 20 minutes. Pork will be fully cooked to at least 145°F in the center and browned when done. Serve warm.

PER SERVING

CALORIES: 161

PROTEIN: 9g

FIBER: 1g

NET CARBOHYDRATES: 3g

FAT: 12g

SODIUM: 416mg

CARBOHYDRATES: 4g

SUGAR: 1g

Avocado Fries

These crispy fries are creamy inside and supercrispy outside.

- **Pantry Staples: None**
- **Hands-On Time: 10 minutes**
- **Cook Time: 6 minutes**

Serves 6

1 large egg

¼ cup coconut flour

2 ounces plain pork rinds, finely crushed

2 medium avocados, peeled, pitted, and sliced into ¼"-thick fries

1 Whisk egg in a medium bowl. Place coconut flour and pork rinds in two separate medium bowls. Dip 1 avocado slice into egg, then coat in coconut flour. Dip in egg once more, then press gently into pork rinds to coat on both sides. Repeat with remaining avocado slices.

2 Place slices into ungreased air fryer basket. Adjust the temperature to 400°F and set the timer for 6 minutes, turning "fries" halfway through. Fries will be crispy on the outside and soft inside when done. Let cool before serving.

PER SERVING

CALORIES: 161

PROTEIN: 8g

FIBER: 5g

NET CARBOHYDRATES: 2g

FAT: 11g

SODIUM: 173mg

CARBOHYDRATES: 7g

SUGAR: 1g

Spicy Turkey Meatballs

Ground turkey can be swapped out for beef in most recipes, and though it's leaner, it contains a high fat percentage. Pair these meatballs with cauliflower or salad for an easy meal.

- **Pantry Staples: Salt, ground black pepper, paprika**
- **Hands-On Time: 10 minutes**
- **Cook Time: 15 minutes**

Yields 18 meatballs

1 pound 85/15 ground turkey
1 large egg, whisked
¼ cup sriracha hot chili sauce
½ teaspoon salt
½ teaspoon paprika
¼ teaspoon ground black pepper

1 Combine all ingredients in a large bowl. Roll mixture into eighteen meatballs, about 3 tablespoons each.

2 Place meatballs into ungreased air fryer basket. Adjust the temperature to 375°F and set the timer for 15 minutes, shaking the basket three times during cooking. Meatballs will be done when browned and internal temperature is at least 165°F. Serve warm.

PER SERVING (3 MEATBALLS)

CALORIES: 146	FAT: 9g
PROTEIN: 13g	SODIUM: 434mg
FIBER: 0g	CARBOHYDRATES: 2g
NET CARBOHYDRATES: 2g	SUGAR: 2g

Crispy Salami Roll-Ups

These roll-ups can be made and placed in the refrigerator for up to 3 days. Just pop them into the air fryer and reheat at 350°F for 1 minute when you're ready to enjoy them.

- **Pantry Staples: None**
- **Hands-On Time: 5 minutes**
- **Cook Time: 4 minutes**

Yields 16 roll-ups

4 ounces cream cheese, broken into 16 equal pieces
16 (0.5-ounce) deli slices Genoa salami

1 Place a piece of cream cheese at the edge of a slice of salami and roll to close. Secure with a toothpick. Repeat with remaining cream cheese pieces and salami.

2 Place roll-ups in an ungreased 6″ round nonstick baking dish and place into air fryer basket. Adjust the temperature to 350°F and set the timer for 4 minutes. Salami will be crispy and cream cheese will be warm when done. Let cool 5 minutes before serving.

PER SERVING (4 ROLL-UPS)

CALORIES: 269	FAT: 22g
PROTEIN: 11g	SODIUM: 1,064mg
FIBER: 0g	CARBOHYDRATES: 2g
NET CARBOHYDRATES: 2g	SUGAR: 1g

Parmesan Zucchini Fries

If you've been afraid of soggy zucchini fries, fear no more! The salt in this recipe draws out moisture from the zucchini, which helps it get nice and crispy in the air fryer. These fries will taste great dipped in low-carb ketchup or your favorite sauce.

- **Pantry Staples: Salt**
- **Hands-On Time: 2 hours 10 minutes**
- **Cook Time: 10 minutes**

Serves 8

2 medium zucchini, ends removed, quartered lengthwise, and sliced into 3"-long fries

½ teaspoon salt

⅓ cup heavy whipping cream

½ cup blanched finely ground almond flour

¾ cup grated Parmesan cheese

1 teaspoon Italian seasoning

1 Sprinkle zucchini with salt and wrap in a kitchen towel to draw out excess moisture. Let sit 2 hours.

2 Pour cream into a medium bowl. In a separate medium bowl, whisk together flour, Parmesan, and Italian seasoning.

3 Place each zucchini fry into cream, then gently shake off excess. Press each fry into dry mixture, coating each side, then place into ungreased air fryer basket. Adjust the temperature to 400°F and set the timer for 10 minutes, turning fries halfway through cooking. Fries will be golden and crispy when done. Place on clean parchment sheet to cool 5 minutes before serving.

PER SERVING

CALORIES: 124
PROTEIN: 5g
FIBER: 1g
NET CARBOHYDRATES: 3g

FAT: 10g
SODIUM: 322mg
CARBOHYDRATES: 4g
SUGAR: 2g

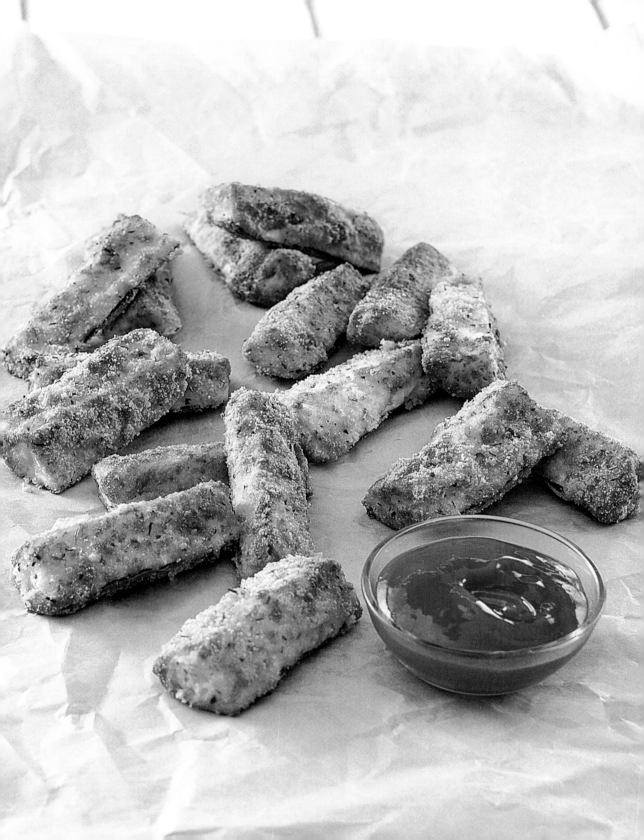

Fried Ranch Pickles

This appetizer is crispy around the edges and full of delicious ranch flavor. The tang from the pickles makes the perfect complement to the breading, which has just a hint of cheese. Serve with a side of additional ranch dressing for dipping.

- **Pantry Staples: None**
- **Hands-On Time: 40 minutes**
- **Cook Time: 10 minutes**

Serves 4

4 dill pickle spears, halved lengthwise

¼ cup ranch dressing

½ cup blanched finely ground almond flour

½ cup grated Parmesan cheese

2 tablespoons dry ranch seasoning

1 Wrap spears in a kitchen towel 30 minutes to soak up excess pickle juice.

2 Pour ranch dressing into a medium bowl and add pickle spears. In a separate medium bowl, mix flour, Parmesan, and ranch seasoning.

3 Remove each spear from ranch dressing and shake off excess. Press gently into dry mixture to coat all sides. Place spears into ungreased air fryer basket. Adjust the temperature to 400°F and set the timer for 10 minutes, turning spears three times during cooking. Serve warm.

PER SERVING

CALORIES: 160	**FAT:** 11g
PROTEIN: 7g	**SODIUM:** 893mg
FIBER: 2g	**CARBOHYDRATES:** 8g
NET CARBOHYDRATES: 6g	**SUGAR:** 1g

Bacon-Wrapped Mozzarella Sticks

This snack has gooey melted cheese and crispy bacon—the perfect mix of salty and savory. Flavorful and low-carb, they can be dipped in everything from low-carb marinara to ranch. Sprinkle with your favorite herbs before wrapping in bacon, or brush the bacon with sriracha for a little heat.

- **Pantry Staples: None**
- **Hands-On Time: 12 minutes**
- **Cook Time: 12 minutes**

Serves 6

6 sticks mozzarella string cheese
6 slices sugar-free bacon

1 Place mozzarella sticks on a medium plate, cover, and place into freezer 1 hour until frozen solid.

2 Wrap each mozzarella stick in 1 piece of bacon and secure with a toothpick. Place into ungreased air fryer basket. Adjust the temperature to 400°F and set the timer for 12 minutes, turning sticks once during cooking. Bacon will be crispy when done. Serve warm.

PER SERVING

CALORIES: 123
PROTEIN: 10g
FIBER: 0g
NET CARBOHYDRATES: 0g

FAT: 9g
SODIUM: 368mg
CARBOHYDRATES: 0g
SUGAR: 0g

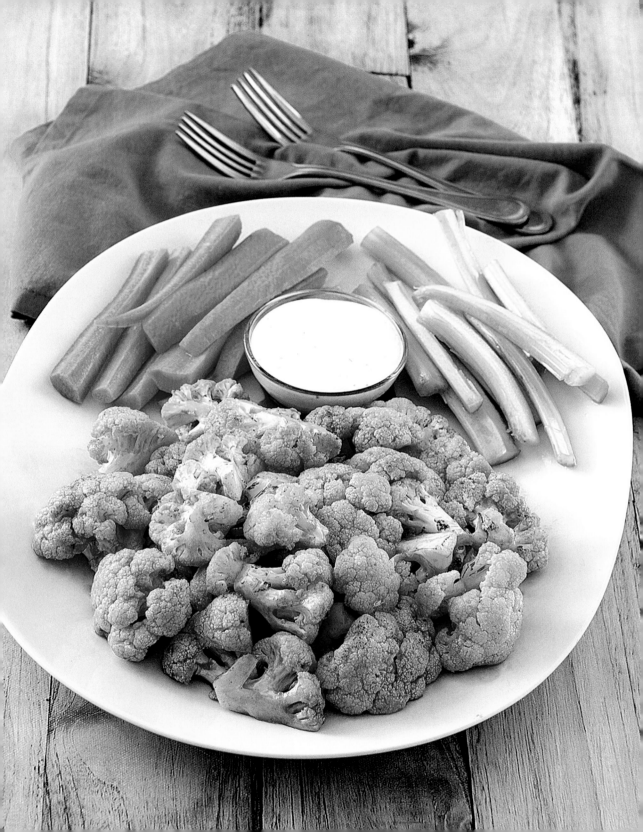

Buffalo Cauliflower Bites

Traditional vegetable platters are a great appetizer, but sometimes they need a little extra flavor to get guests excited. These spicy bites are coated in savory ranch before getting crisped and golden in the air fryer. Serve with ranch for dipping, along with carrots and celery on the side.

- **Pantry Staples: None**
- **Hands-On Time: 5 minutes**
- **Cook Time: 15 minutes**

Serves 6

1 medium head cauliflower, leaves and core removed, cut into bite-sized pieces
4 tablespoons salted butter, melted
¼ cup dry ranch seasoning
⅓ cup buffalo sauce

1 Place cauliflower pieces into a large bowl. Pour butter over cauliflower and toss to coat. Sprinkle in ranch seasoning and toss to coat.

2 Place cauliflower into ungreased air fryer basket. Adjust the temperature to 350°F and set the timer for 12 minutes, shaking the basket three times during cooking.

3 When timer beeps, place cooked cauliflower in a clean large bowl. Toss with buffalo sauce, then return to air fryer basket to cook another 3 minutes. Cauliflower bites will be darkened at the edges and tender when done. Serve warm.

PER SERVING

CALORIES: 112
PROTEIN: 2g
FIBER: 2g
NET CARBOHYDRATES: 7g

FAT: 7g
SODIUM: 1,038mg
CARBOHYDRATES: 9g
SUGAR: 2g

Savory Ranch Chicken Bites

This recipe is perfect for a crowd and doesn't take long to put together. The ranch and cheese melt together to make a creamy sauce for the chicken, which is further complemented by the crispy bacon. Feel free to use your favorite seasoning on the chicken, such as Cajun or buffalo.

- **Pantry Staples: Salt, ground black pepper, coconut oil**
- **Hands-On Time: 10 minutes**
- **Cook Time: 15 minutes**

Serves 6

2 (6-ounce) boneless, skinless chicken breasts, cut into 1" cubes

1 tablespoon coconut oil

½ teaspoon salt

¼ teaspoon ground black pepper

⅓ cup ranch dressing

½ cup shredded Colby cheese

4 slices cooked sugar-free bacon, crumbled

1 Drizzle chicken with coconut oil. Sprinkle with salt and pepper, and place into an ungreased 6" round nonstick baking dish.

2 Place dish into air fryer basket. Adjust the temperature to 370°F and set the timer for 10 minutes, stirring chicken halfway through cooking.

3 When timer beeps, drizzle ranch dressing over chicken and top with Colby and bacon. Adjust the temperature to 400°F and set the timer for 5 minutes. When done, chicken will be browned and have an internal temperature of at least 165°F. Serve warm.

PER SERVING

CALORIES: 164	**FAT:** 9g
PROTEIN: 18g	**SODIUM:** 412mg
FIBER: 0g	**CARBOHYDRATES:** 0g
NET CARBOHYDRATES: 0g	**SUGAR:** 0g

Side Dishes

Sides are an important way to round out main dishes for more complete, satisfying meals. And thanks to the air fryer, whipping up a delicious, nutritious side for any entrée is a snap! With no more than five ingredients and a few minutes of prep time, you can have flavorful, filling sides ready for any occasion.

It is recommended when following a keto diet that most of the carbs you eat come from vegetables, which is why this chapter is full of vegetable-based side recipes that will provide lots of nutrients and perfectly complement your main dishes. And since balance is key to achieving success on the keto diet, you will also find plenty of more indulgent low-carb sides for when those fried-food cravings hit. From Garlic Parmesan–Roasted Cauliflower to Bacon-Jalapeño Cheesy "Breadsticks," this chapter has all the tools you'll need to make easy keto-friendly side dishes!

Baked Jalapeño and Cheese Cauliflower Mash

This dish is the perfect side when you're short on time and ingredients. You likely have most of the ingredients in your refrigerator already. The cream cheese is used as a thickener to give the dish a smooth and creamy texture.

- **Pantry Staples: Salt, ground black pepper**
- **Hands-On Time: 10 minutes**
- **Cook Time: 15 minutes**

Serves 6

1 (12-ounce) steamer bag cauliflower florets, cooked according to package instructions

2 tablespoons salted butter, softened

2 ounces cream cheese, softened

½ cup shredded sharp Cheddar cheese

¼ cup pickled jalapeños

½ teaspoon salt

¼ teaspoon ground black pepper

1 Place cooked cauliflower into a food processor with remaining ingredients. Pulse twenty times until cauliflower is smooth and all ingredients are combined.

2 Spoon mash into an ungreased 6″ round nonstick baking dish. Place dish into air fryer basket. Adjust the temperature to 380°F and set the timer for 15 minutes. The top will be golden brown when done. Serve warm.

PER SERVING

CALORIES: 117	FAT: 9g
PROTEIN: 4g	SODIUM: 390mg
FIBER: 1g	CARBOHYDRATES: 3g
NET CARBOHYDRATES: 2g	SUGAR: 2g

Burger Bun for C

This bun is the perfect quick and easy bread
grilled cheese to breakfast sandwiches. Delic
keep you from reaching for traditional carb-

- **Pantry Staples: Baking powder**
- **Hands-On Time: 2 minutes**
- **Cook Time: 5 minutes**

Serves 1

2 tablespoons salted butter, melted
¼ cup blanched finely ground almond flour
¼ teaspoon baking powder
⅛ teaspoon apple cider vinegar
1 large egg, whisked

OVEN-SAFE BAKING DISHES

You don't have to go out and buy dishes that are specifically made for air fryers. If something is safe for your oven, it's safe for your air fryer! Small ramekins, cake pans, and other mini baking dishes can be used for air frying without a problem.

1   Pou
    Add
    ram
    and

2   Plac
    the
    for
    firm

about 5 minutes, then remove from ramekin
and slice in half. Serve.

PER SERVING

CALORIES: 444	FAT: 41g
PROTEIN: 13g	SODIUM: 374mg
FIBER: 3g	CARBOHYDRATES: 6g
NET CARBOHYDRATES: 3g	SUGAR: 1g

Bacon-Balsa

The sweet balsamic and s
plement just about any
sprouts will surprise

- Pantry St
  black
- Han

...mic Brussels Sprouts

...oky bacon flavors in this recipe make for a dish that can com-
...entrée. Whether you're enjoying chicken or steak, these Brussels
...you with how tasty they are.

...aples: Salt, ground
...epper
...ds-On Time: 5 minutes
...ook Time: 12 minutes

Serves 4

2 cups trimmed and halved
   fresh Brussels sprouts

2 tablespoons olive oil

¼ teaspoon salt

¼ teaspoon ground black
   pepper

2 tablespoons balsamic
   vinegar

2 slices cooked sugar-free
   bacon, crumbled

1. In a large bowl, toss Brussels sprouts in olive oil, then sprinkle with salt and pepper. Place into ungreased air fryer basket. Adjust the temperature to 375°F and set the timer for 12 minutes, shaking the basket halfway through cooking. Brussels sprouts will be tender and browned when done.

2. Place sprouts in a large serving dish and drizzle with balsamic vinegar. Sprinkle bacon over top. Serve warm.

PER SERVING

CALORIES: 112

PROTEIN: 3g

FIBER: 2g

NET CARBOHYDRATES: 3g

FAT: 9g

SODIUM: 254mg

CARBOHYDRATES: 5g

SUGAR: 2g

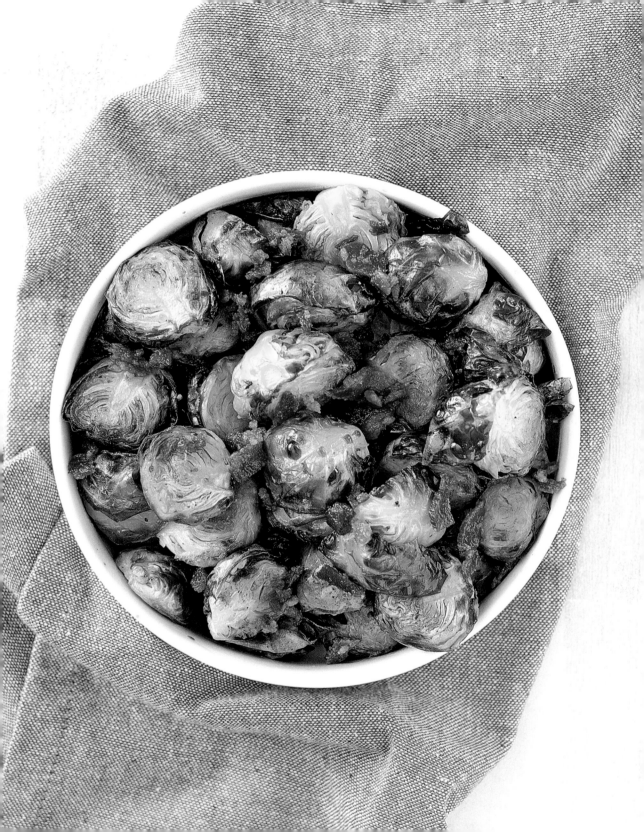

Roasted Asparagus

You don't need much seasoning to give this recipe flavor, as the golden-brown ends add a nice natural sweetness. This dish can be doubled and used for meal prep alongside Butter and Bacon Chicken (see recipe in Chapter 5) or Italian Meatballs (see recipe in Chapter 6) for a well-rounded and delicious spread.

- **Pantry Staples: Salt, ground black pepper**
- **Hands-On Time: 5 minutes**
- **Cook Time: 12 minutes**

Serves 4

1 tablespoon olive oil

1 pound asparagus spears, ends trimmed

¼ teaspoon salt

¼ teaspoon ground black pepper

1 tablespoon salted butter, melted

1 In a large bowl, drizzle olive oil over asparagus spears and sprinkle with salt and pepper.

2 Place spears into ungreased air fryer basket. Adjust the temperature to 375°F and set the timer for 12 minutes, shaking the basket halfway through cooking. Asparagus will be lightly browned and tender when done.

3 Transfer to a large dish and drizzle with butter. Serve warm.

PER SERVING

CALORIES: 73	FAT: 6g
PROTEIN: 2g	SODIUM: 169mg
FIBER: 2g	CARBOHYDRATES: 4g
NET CARBOHYDRATES: 2g	SUGAR: 2g

Cheesy Baked Asparagus

This recipe puts a cheesy spin on simple asparagus. The tender vegetable cooks in a creamy sauce and soaks up all the tasty flavor. Feel free to add ½ teaspoon of your favorite Italian seasoning to really make it pop.

- **Pantry Staples: Salt, ground black pepper**
- **Hands-On Time: 10 minutes**
- **Cook Time: 18 minutes**

Serves 4

½ cup heavy whipping cream

½ cup grated Parmesan cheese

2 ounces cream cheese, softened

1 pound asparagus, ends trimmed, chopped into 1″ pieces

¼ teaspoon salt

¼ teaspoon ground black pepper

1 In a medium bowl, whisk together heavy cream, Parmesan, and cream cheese until combined.

2 Place asparagus into an ungreased 6″ round nonstick baking dish. Pour cheese mixture over top and sprinkle with salt and pepper.

3 Place dish into air fryer basket. Adjust the temperature to 350°F and set the timer for 18 minutes. Asparagus will be tender when done. Serve warm.

PER SERVING

CALORIES: 221	FAT: 18g
PROTEIN: 7g	SODIUM: 435mg
FIBER: 2g	CARBOHYDRATES: 7g
NET CARBOHYDRATES: 5g	SUGAR: 3g

Dijon Roast Cabbage

If you like honey mustard, you'll love the sweet sauce that is drizzled over the crispy cabbage in this dish. It's easy to make, and you may already have most of the ingredients in your pantry. It's a great side to brats or a buttery chicken thigh.

- **Pantry Staples: Salt**
- **Hands-On Time: 10 minutes**
- **Cook Time: 10 minutes**

Serves 4

1 small head cabbage, cored and sliced into 1"-thick slices

2 tablespoons olive oil, divided

½ teaspoon salt

1 tablespoon Dijon mustard

1 teaspoon apple cider vinegar

1 teaspoon granular erythritol

1 Drizzle each cabbage slice with 1 tablespoon olive oil, then sprinkle with salt. Place slices into ungreased air fryer basket, working in batches if needed. Adjust the temperature to 350°F and set the timer for 10 minutes. Cabbage will be tender and edges will begin to brown when done.

2 In a small bowl, whisk remaining olive oil with mustard, vinegar, and erythritol. Drizzle over cabbage in a large serving dish. Serve warm.

PER SERVING

CALORIES: 111

PROTEIN: 3g

FIBER: 4g

NET CARBOHYDRATES: 7g

SUGAR ALCOHOL: 1g

FAT: 7g

SODIUM: 416mg

CARBOHYDRATES: 12g

SUGAR: 6g

Garlic Parmesan–Roasted Cauliflower

As is true of potatoes, there are so many ways to dress up cauliflower. And while a lot of recipes require draining and cooking it twice, this simple recipe gets back to basics through roasting. Made mostly with ingredients you'll have on hand, this easy side goes with just about anything.

- **Pantry Staples: Salt**
- **Hands-On Time: 5 minutes**
- **Cook Time: 15 minutes**

Serves 6

1 medium head cauliflower, leaves and core removed, cut into florets

2 tablespoons salted butter, melted

½ tablespoon salt

2 cloves garlic, peeled and finely minced

½ cup grated Parmesan cheese, divided

1 Toss cauliflower in a large bowl with butter. Sprinkle with salt, garlic, and ¼ cup Parmesan.

2 Place florets into ungreased air fryer basket. Adjust the temperature to 350°F and set the timer for 15 minutes, shaking basket halfway through cooking. Cauliflower will be browned at the edges and tender when done.

3 Transfer florets to a large serving dish and sprinkle with remaining Parmesan. Serve warm.

PER SERVING

CALORIES: 94	FAT: 6g
PROTEIN: 4g	SODIUM: 791mg
FIBER: 2g	CARBOHYDRATES: 6g
NET CARBOHYDRATES: 4g	SUGAR: 2g

Cauliflower Rice Balls

This dish is so delicious it might just steal the show! The rice balls are crunchy on the outside and full of gooey cheese inside—but still loaded with nutrients. Serve as a side or with warmed low-carb marinara and garnished with Parmesan.

- **Pantry Staples:** Salt
- **Hands-On Time:** 10 minutes
- **Cook Time:** 8 minutes

Serves 4

1 (10-ounce) steamer bag cauliflower rice, cooked according to package instructions

½ cup shredded mozzarella cheese

1 large egg

2 ounces plain pork rinds, finely crushed

¼ teaspoon salt

½ teaspoon Italian seasoning

1 Place cauliflower into a large bowl and mix with mozzarella.

2 Whisk egg in a separate medium bowl. Place pork rinds into another large bowl with salt and Italian seasoning.

3 Separate cauliflower mixture into four equal sections and form each into a ball. Carefully dip a ball into whisked egg, then roll in pork rinds. Repeat with remaining balls.

4 Place cauliflower balls into ungreased air fryer basket. Adjust the temperature to 400°F and set the timer for 8 minutes. Rice balls will be golden when done.

5 Use a spatula to carefully move cauliflower balls to a large dish for serving. Serve warm.

PER SERVING

CALORIES: 158

PROTEIN: 15g

FIBER: 2g

NET CARBOHYDRATES: 2g

FAT: 9g

SODIUM: 509mg

CARBOHYDRATES: 4g

SUGAR: 2g

Cheesy Loaded Broccoli

This dish is a favorite of kids and adults alike. It tastes similar to the topping of a loaded baked potato; with all the best parts—like cheese and bacon—no one will even miss the potato!

- **Pantry Staples: Salt, coconut oil**
- **Hands-On Time: 10 minutes**
- **Cook Time: 10 minutes**

Serves 2

3 cups fresh broccoli florets

1 tablespoon coconut oil

¼ teaspoon salt

½ cup shredded sharp Cheddar cheese

¼ cup sour cream

4 slices cooked sugar-free bacon, crumbled

1 medium scallion, trimmed and sliced on the bias

1 Place broccoli into ungreased air fryer basket, drizzle with coconut oil, and sprinkle with salt. Adjust the temperature to 350°F and set the timer for 8 minutes. Shake basket three times during cooking to avoid burned spots.

2 When timer beeps, sprinkle broccoli with Cheddar and set the timer for 2 additional minutes. When done, cheese will be melted and broccoli will be tender.

3 Serve warm in a large serving dish, topped with sour cream, crumbled bacon, and scallion slices.

PER SERVING

CALORIES: 381	**FAT:** 27g
PROTEIN: 19g	**SODIUM:** 917mg
FIBER: 4g	**CARBOHYDRATES:** 11g
NET CARBOHYDRATES: 7g	**SUGAR:** 3g

Buttery Mushrooms

This simple side packs as much flavor as it does health benefits, including Vitamin D. These tender, buttery mushrooms make the perfect side dish to any of your favorite keto entrées.

- **Pantry Staples: Salt, ground black pepper**
- **Hands-On Time: 10 minutes**
- **Cook Time: 10 minutes**

Serves 4

8 ounces cremini mushrooms, halved

2 tablespoons salted butter, melted

¼ teaspoon salt

¼ teaspoon ground black pepper

In a medium bowl, toss mushrooms with butter, then sprinkle with salt and pepper. Place into ungreased air fryer basket. Adjust the temperature to 400°F and set the timer for 10 minutes, shaking the basket halfway through cooking. Mushrooms will be tender when done. Serve warm.

PER SERVING

CALORIES: 63	FAT: 5g
PROTEIN: 1g	SODIUM: 194mg
FIBER: 0g	CARBOHYDRATES: 3g
NET CARBOHYDRATES: 3g	SUGAR: 1g

"Faux-tato" Hash

Raw radishes are often used in salads for a light crunch, but when cooked they take on a whole new flavor that is slightly peppery. This recipe is the perfect addition to any meal one might normally pair with potatoes. You can also add your favorite go-to vegetable seasoning blend for even more flavor.

- **Pantry Staples: ground black pepper, garlic powder**
- **Hands-On Time: 10 minutes**
- **Cook Time: 12 minutes**

Serves 4

1 pound radishes, ends removed, quartered

¼ medium yellow onion, peeled and diced

½ medium green bell pepper, seeded and chopped

2 tablespoons salted butter, melted

½ teaspoon garlic powder

¼ teaspoon ground black pepper

1 In a large bowl, combine radishes, onion, and bell pepper. Toss with butter.

2 Sprinkle garlic powder and black pepper over mixture in bowl, then spoon into ungreased air fryer basket.

3 Adjust the temperature to 320°F and set the timer for 12 minutes. Shake basket halfway through cooking. Radishes will be tender when done. Serve warm.

PER SERVING

CALORIES: 69	FAT: 5g
PROTEIN: 1g	SODIUM: 73mg
FIBER: 2g	CARBOHYDRATES: 4g
NET CARBOHYDRATES: 2g	SUGAR: 2g

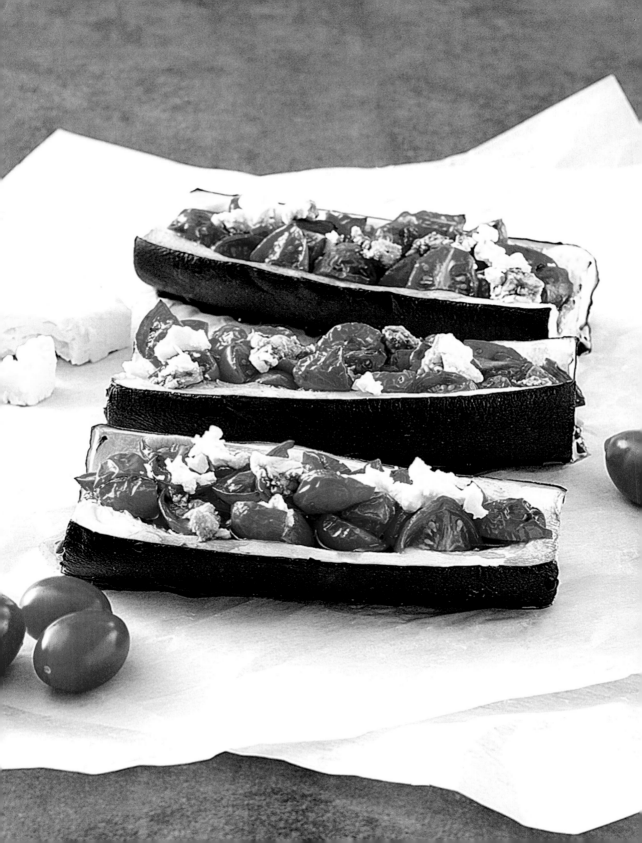

Mediterranean Zucchini Boats

This dish takes advantage of the versatile flavor of zucchini, giving it a Greek-inspired twist. Try adding 2 tablespoons chopped kalamata olives to your filling for a pleasant burst of tangy flavor.

- **Pantry Staples: Salt**
- **Hands-On Time: 5 minutes**
- **Cook Time: 10 minutes**

Serves 4

1 large zucchini, ends removed, halved lengthwise
6 grape tomatoes, quartered
¼ teaspoon salt
¼ cup feta cheese
1 tablespoon balsamic vinegar
1 tablespoon olive oil

1 Use a spoon to scoop out 2 tablespoons from center of each zucchini half, making just enough space to fill with tomatoes and feta.

2 Place tomatoes evenly in centers of zucchini halves and sprinkle with salt. Place into ungreased air fryer basket. Adjust the temperature to 350°F and set the timer for 10 minutes. When done, zucchini will be tender.

3 Transfer boats to a serving tray and sprinkle with feta, then drizzle with vinegar and olive oil. Serve warm.

PER SERVING

CALORIES: 74	FAT: 5g
PROTEIN: 2g	SODIUM: 238mg
FIBER: 1g	CARBOHYDRATES: 4g
NET CARBOHYDRATES: 3g	SUGAR: 3g

Roasted Broccoli Salad

This recipe puts an end to any perceptions that broccoli is boring! Bursting with savory flavors, a little bit of tang, and just the right amount of crunch, this salad is the perfect complement to any dinner.

- Pantry Staples: Salt, ground black pepper
- Hands-On Time: 5 minutes
- Cook Time: 7 minutes

Serves 4

2 cups fresh broccoli florets, chopped
1 tablespoon olive oil
¼ teaspoon salt
⅛ teaspoon ground black pepper
¼ cup lemon juice, divided
¼ cup shredded Parmesan cheese
¼ cup sliced roasted almonds

1 In a large bowl, toss broccoli and olive oil together. Sprinkle with salt and pepper, then drizzle with 2 tablespoons lemon juice.

2 Place broccoli into ungreased air fryer basket. Adjust the temperature to 350°F and set the timer for 7 minutes, shaking the basket halfway through cooking. Broccoli will be golden on the edges when done.

3 Place broccoli into a large serving bowl and drizzle with remaining lemon juice. Sprinkle with Parmesan and almonds. Serve warm.

PER SERVING

CALORIES: 102	FAT: 7g
PROTEIN: 4g	SODIUM: 245mg
FIBER: 2g	CARBOHYDRATES: 6g
NET CARBOHYDRATES: 4g	SUGAR: 1g

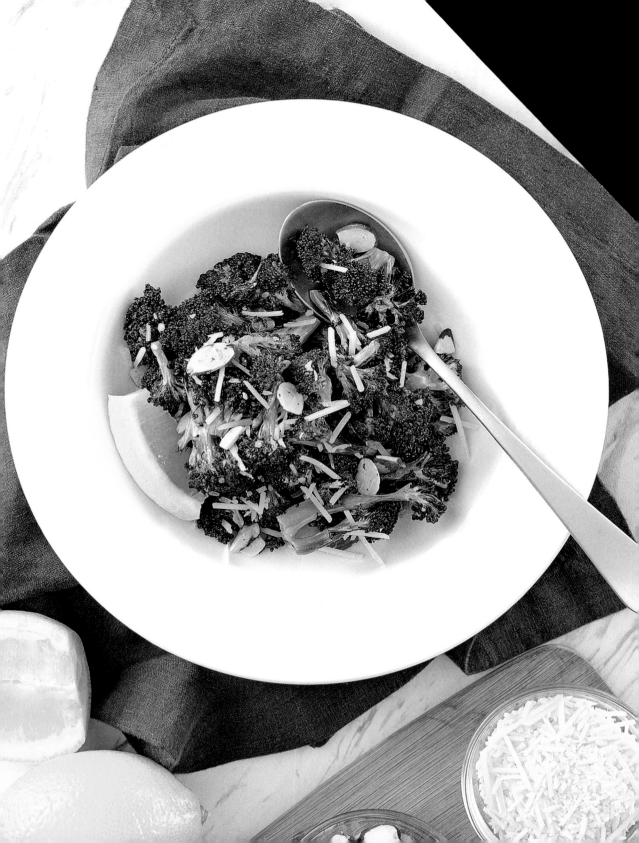

apeño Cheesy
ks"

cipe could fool any carb lover! It's as easy as it seems, and this an entrée, simply add your favorite pizza toppings, such

- **Pantry Staples: None**
- **Hands-On Time: 10 minutes**
- **Cook Time: 15 minutes**

Yields 8 sticks

2 cups shredded mozzarella cheese

¼ cup grated Parmesan cheese

¼ cup chopped pickled jalapeños

2 large eggs, whisked

4 slices cooked sugar-free bacon, chopped

1 Mix all ingredients together in a large bowl. Cut a piece of parchment paper to fit inside air fryer basket.

2 Dampen your hands with a bit of water and press out mixture into a circle to fit on ungreased parchment. You may need to separate into two smaller circles, depending on the size of air fryer.

3 Place parchment with cheese mixture into air fryer basket. Adjust the temperature to 320°F and set the timer for 15 minutes. Carefully flip when 5 minutes remain on timer. The top will be golden brown when done. Slice into eight sticks. Serve warm.

PER SERVING (2 STICKS)

CALORIES: 275	FAT: 16g
PROTEIN: 22g	SODIUM: 783mg
FIBER: 0g	CARBOHYDRATES: 5g
NET CARBOHYDRATES: 5g	SUGAR: 1g

Dinner Rolls

If you're a fan of multigrain rolls, this recipe is for you. The ground flax helps add a wheat-like flavor to the rolls, making them the perfect keto bread replacement. They can also be enjoyed as slider buns, or used with your favorite sandwich toppings.

- **Pantry Staples: Baking powder**
- **Hands-On Time: 10 minutes**
- **Cook Time: 12 minutes**

Serves 6

1 cup shredded mozzarella cheese
1 ounce cream cheese, broken into small pieces
1 cup blanched finely ground almond flour
¼ cup ground flaxseed
½ teaspoon baking powder
1 large egg, whisked

A GO-TO BREAD!

Bookmark this dough recipe for all your bread needs! You can make it into larger buns, or even longer sub rolls for sandwiches. It has a taste similar to a multigrain bread, so feel free to get creative. The temperature should always be set to 320°F, and the cook time will remain the same unless you double the recipe (just add 2 more minutes).

1. Place mozzarella, cream cheese, and flour in a large microwave-safe bowl. Microwave on high 1 minute. Mix until smooth.

2. Add flaxseed, baking powder, and egg to mixture until fully combined and smooth. Microwave an additional 15 seconds if dough becomes too firm.

3. Separate dough into six equal pieces and roll each into a ball. Place rolls into ungreased air fryer basket. Adjust the temperature to 320°F and set the timer for 12 minutes, turning rolls halfway through cooking. Allow rolls to cool completely before serving, about 5 minutes.

PER SERVING

CALORIES: 235	FAT: 18g
PROTEIN: 11g	SODIUM: 199mg
FIBER: 4g	CARBOHYDRATES: 7g
NET CARBOHYDRATES: 3g	SUGAR: 1g

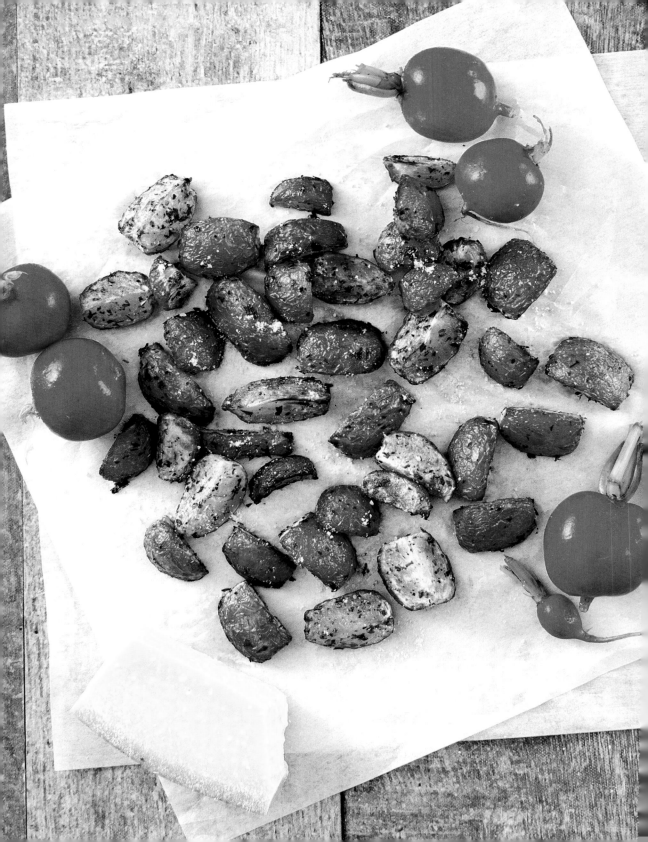

Parmesan Herb Radishes

While most root vegetables have too many carbs to easily fit into a ketogenic diet, radishes have only about 2 grams of net carbs per cup. When cooked, radishes take on a slight peppery flavor and have a tender bite that serves as a nice texture alternative to potatoes.

- **Pantry Staples: ground black pepper, garlic powder**
- **Hands-On Time: 10 minutes**
- **Cook Time: 10 minutes**

Serves 6

1 pound radishes, ends removed, quartered
2 tablespoons salted butter, melted
½ teaspoon garlic powder
½ teaspoon dried parsley
¼ teaspoon dried oregano
¼ teaspoon ground black pepper
¼ cup grated Parmesan cheese

1 Place radishes into a medium bowl and drizzle with butter. Sprinkle with garlic powder, parsley, oregano, and pepper, then place into ungreased air fryer basket. Adjust the temperature to 350°F and set the timer for 10 minutes, shaking the basket three times during cooking. Radishes will be done when tender and golden.

2 Place radishes into a large serving dish and sprinkle with Parmesan. Serve warm.

PER SERVING

CALORIES: 59		FAT: 5g	
PROTEIN: 2g		SODIUM: 124mg	
FIBER: 1g		CARBOHYDRATES: 3g	
NET CARBOHYDRATES: 2g		SUGAR: 1g	

ngs

usually coated with carb-filled bread crumbs or flour. This
crunchy exterior you know and love with the best low-carb
pork rinds! These rings taste great on their own, but can also

- **Pantry Staples: None**
- **Hands-On Time: 10 minutes**
- **Cook Time: 5 minutes**

Serves 8

1 large egg
¼ cup coconut flour
2 ounces plain pork rinds,
    finely crushed
1 large white onion, peeled
    and sliced into 8 (¼") rings

PORK RIND DIFFERENCES

Not all pork rinds are created
equal, and some are loaded with
unnecessary ingredients like MSG
and maltodextrin. Simply read
labels to choose higher-quality
pork rinds with fewer ingredients
for the best flavor and crunch.

1 Whisk egg in a medium bowl. Place coconut
flour and pork rinds in two separate medium
bowls. Dip each onion ring into egg, then
coat in coconut flour. Dip coated onion ring
in egg once more, then press gently into
pork rinds to cover all sides.

2 Place rings into ungreased air fryer basket.
Adjust the temperature to 400°F and set
the timer for 5 minutes, turning the onion
rings halfway through cooking. Onion rings
will be golden and crispy when done. Serve
warm.

PER SERVING

CALORIES: 79	FAT: 3g
PROTEIN: 6g	SODIUM: 129mg
FIBER: 2g	CARBOHYDRATES: 6g
NET CARBOHYDRATES: 4g	SUGAR: 2g

Crispy Green Beans

The air fryer allows green beans to retain more vitamins and flavor, as opposed to boiling, which removes a lot of the nutrients and can make the green beans taste watery. This dish tastes great with an extra drizzle of butter, or accompanied by Caesar salad dressing for dipping.

- **Pantry Staples: Salt, ground black pepper**
- **Hands-On Time: 5 minutes**
- **Cook Time: 8 minutes**

Serves 4

2 teaspoons olive oil
½ pound fresh green beans, ends trimmed
¼ teaspoon salt
¼ teaspoon ground black pepper

1. In a large bowl, drizzle olive oil over green beans and sprinkle with salt and pepper.

2. Place green beans into ungreased air fryer basket. Adjust the temperature to 350°F and set the timer for 8 minutes, shaking the basket two times during cooking. Green beans will be dark golden and crispy at the edges when done. Serve warm.

PER SERVING

CALORIES: 37	FAT: 2g
PROTEIN: 1g	SODIUM: 148mg
FIBER: 2g	CARBOHYDRATES: 4g
NET CARBOHYDRATES: 2g	SUGAR: 2g

LEGUMES ON THE KETO DIET
While some following a ketogenic diet may choose not to eat legumes, others utilize a more flexible dieting style that allows certain legumes in moderation. Legumes are loaded with nutrients like folate and can be a great addition to your meal planning if you decide to include them in your own keto goals.

Flatbread Dippers

If you're enjoying a creamy soup or dip, the perfect side dish is a crunchy dipper to help you savor every last bite. These Flatbread Dippers are similar to a thin flatbread and have a mild flavor that won't overpower your entrée. And with just three ingredients, you can whip them up in less than 15 minutes!

- **Pantry Staples: None**
- **Hands-On Time: 5 minutes**
- **Cook Time: 8 minutes**

Yields 12 triangles

1 cup shredded mozzarella cheese

1 ounce cream cheese, broken into small pieces

½ cup blanched finely ground almond flour

1 Place mozzarella into a large microwave-safe bowl. Add cream cheese pieces. Microwave on high 60 seconds, then stir to combine. Add flour and stir until a soft ball of dough forms.

2 Cut dough ball into two equal pieces. Cut a piece of parchment to fit into air fryer basket. Press each dough piece into a 5" round on ungreased parchment.

3 Place parchment with dough into air fryer basket. Adjust the temperature to 350°F and set the timer for 8 minutes. Carefully flip the flatbread over halfway through cooking. Flatbread will be golden brown when done.

4 Let flatbread cool 5 minutes, then slice each round into six triangles. Serve warm.

PER SERVING (3 TRIANGLES)

CALORIES: 194	**FAT:** 15g
PROTEIN: 10g	**SODIUM:** 218mg
FIBER: 2g	**CARBOHYDRATES:** 4g
NET CARBOHYDRATES: 2g	**SUGAR:** 1g

Mini Spinach and Sweet Pepper Poppers

These are an excellent alternative to jalapeño poppers, especially if spicy isn't your thing. They're just a little sweet but pack a big crunch that pairs perfectly with the creamy garlic filling. The spinach is an easy way to get in your leafy greens, but feel free to omit if you prefer.

- **Pantry Staples: Garlic powder**
- **Hands-On Time: 10 minutes**
- **Cook Time: 8 minutes**

Yields 16 poppers

4 ounces cream cheese, softened

1 cup chopped fresh spinach leaves

½ teaspoon garlic powder

8 mini sweet bell peppers, tops removed, seeded, and halved lengthwise

1 In a medium bowl, mix cream cheese, spinach, and garlic powder. Place 1 tablespoon mixture into each sweet pepper half and press down to smooth.

2 Place poppers into ungreased air fryer basket. Adjust the temperature to 400°F and set the timer for 8 minutes. Poppers will be done when cheese is browned on top and peppers are tender-crisp. Serve warm.

PER SERVING (4 POPPERS)

CALORIES: 116

PROTEIN: 3g

FIBER: 1g

NET CARBOHYDRATES: 4g

FAT: 8g

SODIUM: 109mg

CARBOHYDRATES: 5g

SUGAR: 3g

Roasted Brussels Sprouts

When you roast vegetables, it brings out their natural sweetness—and that's no different for Brussels sprouts. This easy dish comes together in just a few minutes, and the caramelized, crispy edges of the leaves and tender insides will make this a staple side to any protein.

- **Pantry Staples: Salt, ground black pepper, garlic powder, coconut oil**
- **Hands-On Time: 5 minutes**
- **Cook Time: 10 minutes**

Serves 6

1 pound fresh Brussels sprouts, trimmed and halved
2 tablespoons coconut oil
½ teaspoon salt
¼ teaspoon ground black pepper
½ teaspoon garlic powder
1 tablespoon salted butter, melted

1 Place Brussels sprouts into a large bowl. Drizzle with coconut oil and sprinkle with salt, pepper, and garlic powder.

2 Place Brussels sprouts into ungreased air fryer basket. Adjust the temperature to 350°F and set the timer for 10 minutes, shaking the basket three times during cooking. Brussels sprouts will be dark golden and tender when done.

3 Place cooked sprouts in a large serving dish and drizzle with butter. Serve warm.

PER SERVING

CALORIES: 89	FAT: 6g
PROTEIN: 3g	SODIUM: 227mg
FIBER: 3g	CARBOHYDRATES: 7g
NET CARBOHYDRATES: 4g	SUGAR: 2g

Roasted Salsa

Air fryers are a great way to cook a meal without heating up your living area (like a conventional oven often does). During the warmer months, when tomatoes are in season, this salsa makes an especially delicious topping to chicken thighs, taco bowls, or eggs.

- **Pantry Staples: Salt, coconut oil**
- **Hands-On Time: 5 minutes**
- **Cook Time: 30 minutes**

Yields 2 cups

2 large San Marzano tomatoes, cored and cut into large chunks

½ medium white onion, peeled and large-diced

½ medium jalapeño, seeded and large-diced

2 cloves garlic, peeled and diced

½ teaspoon salt

1 tablespoon coconut oil

¼ cup fresh lime juice

MAKE IT SPICY!

If you're a fan of spicy salsa, feel free to add more jalapeños, or sub in your favorite spicy pepper. Serranos and habaneros offer more heat than jalapeños and have great flavor. You can also add ¼ teaspoon cayenne pepper to the finished salsa for an extra kick.

1 Place tomatoes, onion, and jalapeño into an ungreased 6″ round nonstick baking dish. Add garlic, then sprinkle with salt and drizzle with coconut oil.

2 Place dish into air fryer basket. Adjust the temperature to 300°F and set the timer for 30 minutes. Vegetables will be dark brown around the edges and tender when done.

3 Pour mixture into a food processor or blender. Add lime juice. Process on low speed 30 seconds until only a few chunks remain.

4 Transfer salsa to a sealable container and refrigerate at least 1 hour. Serve chilled.

PER SERVING (¼ CUP)

CALORIES: 28	FAT: 2g
PROTEIN: 1g	SODIUM: 148mg
FIBER: 1g	CARBOHYDRATES: 3g
NET CARBOHYDRATES: 2g	SUGAR: 2g

5

Chicken Main Dishes

Chicken is a great protein to keep on hand—especially when following a keto diet. It's extremely versatile, inexpensive, and absolutely delicious. Plus, it is full of healthy protein. From ground chicken thighs to wings to even an entire bird, any part of the chicken can be turned into a delectable main dish with the air fryer.

This chapter is full of easy keto chicken recipes for your whole family, from Chicken Fajita Poppers to Chipotle Drumsticks. With just a few ingredients and your air fryer, you can have a satisfying meal on the table in no time. So let's get cooking!

Salt and Pepper Wings

Sauces and rubs are delicious, but don't underestimate the power of simple flavors. These wings are extra crunchy and work great for meal prep, since they remain crispy when reheated. Feel free to pair them with your favorite sauce, such as low-carb barbecue or buttermilk ranch.

- **Pantry Staples: Salt, ground black pepper**
- **Hands-On Time: 5 minutes**
- **Cook Time: 25 minutes**

Serves 4

2 pounds bone-in chicken wings, separated at joints
1 teaspoon salt
½ teaspoon ground black pepper

MEAL PREP WINGS

Make a batch of these wings at the beginning of the week, then simply reheat them in the air fryer at 400°F for 5 minutes. Also feel free to toss them in garlic butter or buffalo sauce, or sprinkle with lemon pepper seasoning once reheated.

1 Sprinkle wings with salt and pepper, then place into ungreased air fryer basket in a single layer, working in batches if needed.

2 Adjust the temperature to 400°F and set the timer for 25 minutes, shaking the basket every 7 minutes during cooking. Wings should have an internal temperature of at least 165°F and be golden brown when done. Serve warm.

PER SERVING

CALORIES: 316
PROTEIN: 29g
FIBER: 0g
NET CARBOHYDRATES: 0g
FAT: 22g
SODIUM: 720mg
CARBOHYDRATES: 0g
SUGAR: 0g

Garlic Dill Wings

Made mostly with pantry staples, this recipe is great when you need a last-minute meal that won't be short on flavor. The dill brightens up the wings to create a flavor that reminds you of ranch mix. These wings pair well with a tangy Greek yogurt–based sauce such as tzatziki for dipping.

- **Pantry Staples: Salt, ground black pepper, garlic powder**
- **Hands-On Time: 5 minutes**
- **Cook Time: 25 minutes**

Serves 4

2 pounds bone-in chicken wings, separated at joints
½ teaspoon salt
½ teaspoon ground black pepper
½ teaspoon onion powder
½ teaspoon garlic powder
1 teaspoon dried dill

1 In a large bowl, toss wings with salt, pepper, onion powder, garlic powder, and dill until evenly coated. Place wings into ungreased air fryer basket in a single layer, working in batches if needed.

2 Adjust the temperature to 400°F and set the timer for 25 minutes, shaking the basket every 7 minutes during cooking. Wings should have an internal temperature of at least 165°F and be golden brown when done. Serve warm.

PER SERVING

CALORIES: 319	FAT: 22g
PROTEIN: 29g	SODIUM: 430mg
FIBER: 0g	CARBOHYDRATES: 1g
NET CARBOHYDRATES: 1g	SUGAR: 0g

Chicken Fajita Poppers

These poppers are not only delicious and easy to make, but they also reheat easily in the microwave in just 1 minute on high, making them perfect for meal prep. To add more fat and flavor to this meal, simply pair with your favorite dipping sauce such as sour cream or guacamole.

- Pantry Staples: None
- Hands-On Time: 10 minutes
- Cook Time: 20 minutes

Yields 18 poppers

1 pound ground chicken thighs

½ medium green bell pepper, seeded and finely chopped

¼ medium yellow onion, peeled and finely chopped

½ cup shredded pepper jack cheese

1 (1-ounce) packet gluten-free fajita seasoning

PREMADE SEASONING

Many premade seasonings have additives like maltodextrin, sugar, or flour. There are, however, a growing number of keto-friendly options on the market. Just read labels before making any purchases.

1 In a large bowl, combine all ingredients. Form mixture into eighteen 2″ balls and place in a single layer into ungreased air fryer basket, working in batches if needed.

2 Adjust the temperature to 350°F and set the timer for 20 minutes. Carefully use tongs to turn poppers halfway through cooking. When 5 minutes remain on timer, increase temperature to 400°F to give the poppers a dark golden-brown color. Shake air fryer basket once more when 2 minutes remain on timer. Serve warm.

PER SERVING (3 POPPERS)

CALORIES: 164	FAT: 8g
PROTEIN: 16g	SODIUM: 397mg
FIBER: 0g	CARBOHYDRATES: 5g
NET CARBOHYDRATES: 5g	SUGAR: 0g

Chicken Pesto Pizzas

When you think of ground meat, you may first think of beef and turkey. But don't forget about ground chicken! It is the perfect mild canvas for a variety of flavors. The pairing of chicken and pesto in this recipe is mouthwateringly delicious and won't make you feel lethargic.

- **Pantry Staples: Salt, ground black pepper**
- **Hands-On Time: 10 minutes**
- **Cook Time: 12 minutes**

Serves 4

1 pound ground chicken thighs
¼ teaspoon salt
⅛ teaspoon ground black pepper
¼ cup basil pesto
1 cup shredded mozzarella cheese
4 grape tomatoes, sliced

BUYING GROUND CHICKEN

You can usually find ground chicken right next to the other precut chicken portions at your local store, but if you have trouble, try asking the butcher. They can even grind some up for you fresh if they don't normally carry it pre-packaged. You can also use a meat grinder at home to make your own.

1 Cut four squares of parchment paper to fit into your air fryer basket.

2 Place ground chicken in a large bowl and mix with salt and pepper. Divide mixture into four equal sections.

3 Wet your hands with water to prevent sticking, then press each section into a 6" circle onto a piece of ungreased parchment. Place each chicken crust into air fryer basket, working in batches if needed.

4 Adjust the temperature to 350°F and set the timer for 10 minutes, turning crusts halfway through cooking.

5 When the timer beeps, spread 1 tablespoon pesto across the top of each crust, then sprinkle with ¼ cup mozzarella and top with 1 sliced tomato. Continue cooking at 350°F for 2 minutes. Cheese will be melted and brown when done. Serve warm.

PER SERVING

CALORIES: 318	**FAT:** 19g
PROTEIN: 28g	**SODIUM:** 546mg
FIBER: 0g	**CARBOHYDRATES:** 4g
NET CARBOHYDRATES: 4g	**SUGAR:** 2g

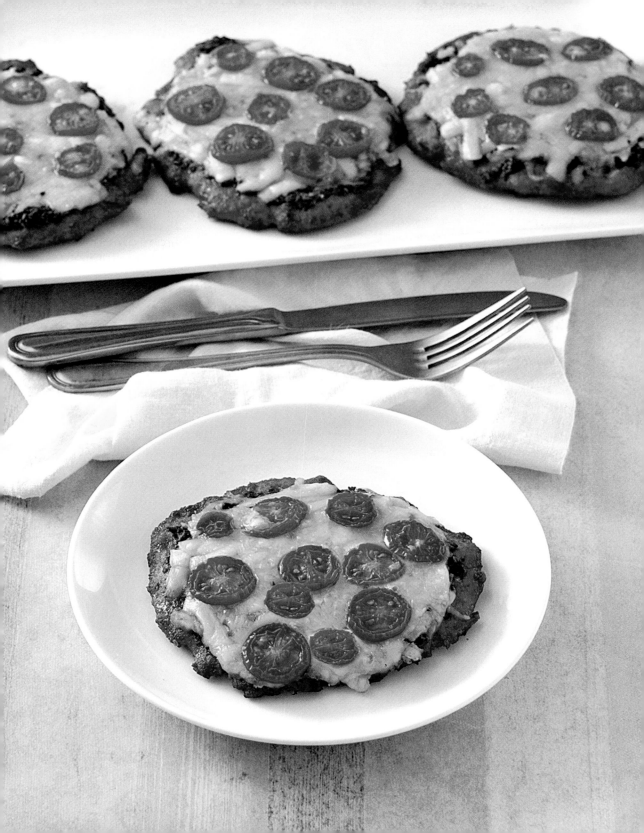

Broccoli and Cheese–Stuffed Chicken

Chicken breast meat is low in fat and as such can easily get dried out, but the mayonnaise used in this dish seals in moisture. Double this meal for leftovers and reheat in the air fryer at 370°F for 8 minutes.

- **Pantry Staples: Salt, ground black pepper, garlic powder**
- **Hands-On Time: 15 minutes**
- **Cook Time: 20 minutes**

Serves 4

2 ounces cream cheese, softened

1 cup chopped fresh broccoli, steamed

½ cup shredded sharp Cheddar cheese

4 (6-ounce) boneless, skinless chicken breasts

2 tablespoons mayonnaise

¼ teaspoon salt

¼ teaspoon garlic powder

⅛ teaspoon ground black pepper

1 In a medium bowl, combine cream cheese, broccoli, and Cheddar. Cut a 4" pocket into each chicken breast. Evenly divide mixture between chicken breasts; stuff the pocket of each chicken breast with the mixture.

2 Spread ¼ tablespoon mayonnaise per side of each chicken breast, then sprinkle both sides of breasts with salt, garlic powder, and pepper.

3 Place stuffed chicken breasts into ungreased air fryer basket so that the open seams face up. Adjust the temperature to 350°F and set the timer for 20 minutes, turning chicken halfway through cooking. When done, chicken will be golden and have an internal temperature of at least 165°F. Serve warm.

PER SERVING

CALORIES: 364	FAT: 16g
PROTEIN: 43g	SODIUM: 415mg
FIBER: 1g	CARBOHYDRATES: 3g
NET CARBOHYDRATES: 2g	SUGAR: 1g

Pickle-Brined Fried Chicken

The crispy outer coating in this dish is the perfect contrast to the juicy insides, making it a great comfort-food meal for any day. You can also chop the chicken into 2″ cubes before coating to make bite-sized crispy nuggets—simply reduce the cook time to 12 minutes.

- **Pantry Staples: Salt, ground black pepper**
- **Hands-On Time: 1 hour 15 minutes**
- **Cook Time: 20 minutes**

Serves 4

4 (4-ounce) boneless, skinless chicken thighs

⅓ cup dill pickle juice

1 large egg

2 ounces plain pork rinds, crushed

½ teaspoon salt

¼ teaspoon ground black pepper

1 Place chicken thighs in a large sealable bowl or bag and pour pickle juice over them. Place sealed bowl or bag into refrigerator and allow to marinate at least 1 hour up to overnight.

2 In a small bowl, whisk egg. Place pork rinds in a separate medium bowl.

3 Remove chicken thighs from marinade. Shake off excess pickle juice and pat thighs dry with a paper towel. Sprinkle with salt and pepper.

4 Dip each thigh into egg and gently shake off excess. Press into pork rinds to coat each side. Place thighs into ungreased air fryer basket. Adjust the temperature to 400°F and set the timer for 20 minutes. When chicken thighs are done, they will be golden and crispy on the outside with an internal temperature of at least 165°F. Serve warm.

PER SERVING

CALORIES: 344
PROTEIN: 44g
FIBER: 0g
NET CARBOHYDRATES: 0g

FAT: 16g
SODIUM: 711mg
CARBOHYDRATES: 0g
SUGAR: 0g

Spice-Rubbed Chicken Thighs

You don't need traditional breading to get crispy chicken—the skin alone can become ultracrispy in the air fryer. The fat in the skin helps it crisp up, while the rest of the chicken stays juicy. The brightness and energizing flavor from the lime juice makes the entire dish.

- **Pantry Staples: Salt, paprika, garlic powder**
- **Hands-On Time: 10 minutes**
- **Cook Time: 25 minutes**

Serves 4

4 (4-ounce) bone-in, skin-on chicken thighs
½ teaspoon salt
½ teaspoon garlic powder
2 teaspoons chili powder
1 teaspoon paprika
1 teaspoon ground cumin
1 small lime, halved

1 Pat chicken thighs dry and sprinkle with salt, garlic powder, chili powder, paprika, and cumin.

2 Squeeze juice from ½ lime over thighs. Place thighs into ungreased air fryer basket. Adjust the temperature to 380°F and set the timer for 25 minutes, turning thighs halfway through cooking. Thighs will be crispy and browned with an internal temperature of at least 165°F when done.

3 Transfer thighs to a large serving plate and drizzle with remaining lime juice. Serve warm.

PER SERVING

CALORIES: 255	**FAT:** 10g
PROTEIN: 34g	**SODIUM:** 475mg
FIBER: 1g	**CARBOHYDRATES:** 2g
NET CARBOHYDRATES: 1g	**SUGAR:** 0g

Spicy Pork Rind Fried Chicken

This dish is perfect for those who love a bit of heat. Feel free to prep step 1 in the morning before you head out for the day to save time. For leftovers, reheat quickly in the air fryer at 400°F for 8 minutes to get back that crispy crust.

- **Pantry Staples: Ground black pepper, paprika, garlic powder**
- **Hands-On Time: 40 minutes**
- **Cook Time: 20 minutes**

Serves 4

¼ cup buffalo sauce

4 (4-ounce) boneless, skinless chicken breasts

½ teaspoon paprika

½ teaspoon garlic powder

¼ teaspoon ground black pepper

2 ounces plain pork rinds, finely crushed

1 Pour buffalo sauce into a large sealable bowl or bag. Add chicken and toss to coat. Place sealed bowl or bag into refrigerator and let marinate at least 30 minutes up to overnight.

2 Remove chicken from marinade but do not shake excess sauce off chicken. Sprinkle both sides of thighs with paprika, garlic powder, and pepper.

3 Place pork rinds into a large bowl and press each chicken breast into pork rinds to coat evenly on both sides.

4 Place chicken into ungreased air fryer basket. Adjust the temperature to 400°F and set the timer for 20 minutes, turning chicken halfway through cooking. Chicken will be golden and have an internal temperature of at least 165°F when done. Serve warm.

PER SERVING

CALORIES: 185
PROTEIN: 27g
FIBER: 0g
NET CARBOHYDRATES: 1g

FAT: 7g
SODIUM: 731mg
CARBOHYDRATES: 1g
SUGAR: 0g

Chipotle Drumsticks

These deep-red drumsticks pack a huge flavor punch. They're smoky with a bit of tang, similar to a chipotle-inspired barbecue sauce. They're also great for meal prep and last in the refrigerator for up to 5 days.

- **Pantry Staples: Salt, ground black pepper, garlic powder**
- **Hands-On Time: 5 minutes**
- **Cook Time: 25 minutes**

Serves 4

1 tablespoon tomato paste
½ teaspoon chipotle powder
¼ teaspoon apple cider vinegar
¼ teaspoon garlic powder
8 chicken drumsticks
½ teaspoon salt
⅛ teaspoon ground black pepper

1 In a small bowl, combine tomato paste, chipotle powder, vinegar, and garlic powder.

2 Sprinkle drumsticks with salt and pepper, then place into a large bowl and pour in tomato paste mixture. Toss or stir to evenly coat all drumsticks in mixture.

3 Place drumsticks into ungreased air fryer basket. Adjust the temperature to 400°F and set the timer for 25 minutes, turning drumsticks halfway through cooking. Drumsticks will be dark red with an internal temperature of at least 165°F when done. Serve warm.

PER SERVING

CALORIES: 432
PROTEIN: 48g
FIBER: 0g
NET CARBOHYDRATES: 1g

FAT: 22g
SODIUM: 623mg
CARBOHYDRATES: 1g
SUGAR: 0g

Garlic Parmesan Drumsticks

Drumsticks are budget friendly and full of flavor. These dark-golden Garlic Parmesan Drumsticks are coated in a light, buttery sauce but never lose that delicious crispy skin. It's a meal the whole family will love.

- **Pantry Staples: Salt, ground black pepper, garlic powder**
- **Hands-On Time: 5 minutes**
- **Cook Time: 25 minutes**

Serves 4

8 (4-ounce) chicken drumsticks

½ teaspoon salt

⅛ teaspoon ground black pepper

½ teaspoon garlic powder

2 tablespoons salted butter, melted

½ cup grated Parmesan cheese

1 tablespoon dried parsley

1 Sprinkle drumsticks with salt, pepper, and garlic powder. Place drumsticks into ungreased air fryer basket.

2 Adjust the temperature to 400°F and set the timer for 25 minutes, turning drumsticks halfway through cooking. Drumsticks will be golden and have an internal temperature of at least 165°F when done.

3 Transfer drumsticks to a large serving dish. Pour butter over drumsticks, and sprinkle with Parmesan and parsley. Serve warm.

PER SERVING

CALORIES: 533	FAT: 30g
PROTEIN: 52g	SODIUM: 845mg
FIBER: 0g	CARBOHYDRATES: 3g
NET CARBOHYDRATES: 3g	SUGAR: 0g

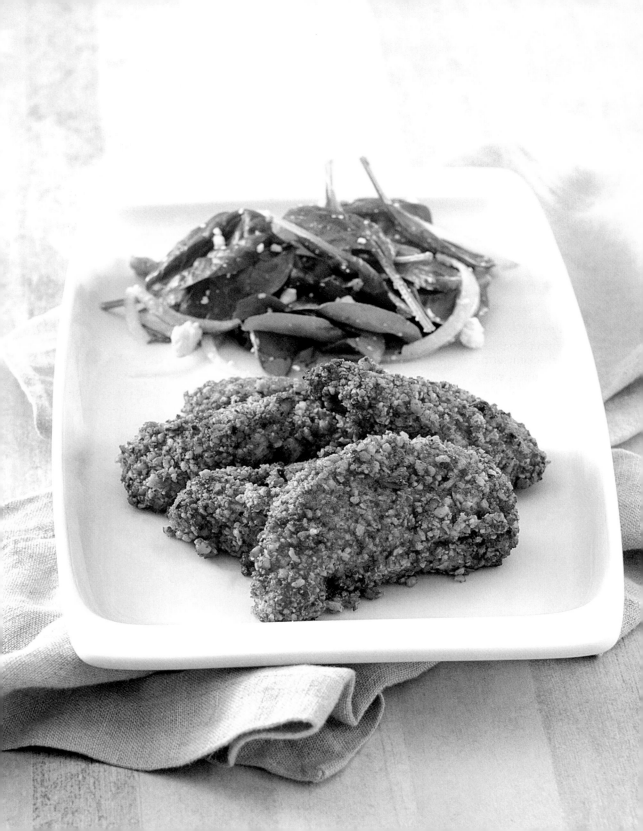

Pecan-Crusted Chicken Tenders

Pecans are an excellent source of fat and great to enjoy in moderation when on a keto diet. They can be sweet but also pair well with more savory sauces like those made with Dijon mustard. Round out the meal with a crisp green salad.

- **Pantry Staples: Salt, ground black pepper**
- **Hands-On Time: 10 minutes**
- **Cook Time: 12 minutes**

Serves 4

2 tablespoons mayonnaise

1 teaspoon Dijon mustard

1 pound boneless, skinless chicken tenders

½ teaspoon salt

¼ teaspoon ground black pepper

½ cup chopped roasted pecans, finely ground

1 In a small bowl, whisk mayonnaise and mustard until combined. Brush mixture onto chicken tenders on both sides, then sprinkle tenders with salt and pepper.

2 Place pecans in a medium bowl and press each tender into pecans to coat each side.

3 Place tenders into ungreased air fryer basket in a single layer, working in batches if needed. Adjust the temperature to 375°F and set the timer for 12 minutes, turning tenders halfway through cooking. Tenders will be golden brown and have an internal temperature of at least 165°F when done. Serve warm.

PER SERVING

CALORIES: 237
PROTEIN: 22g
FIBER: 1g
NET CARBOHYDRATES: 1g

FAT: 15g
SODIUM: 469mg
CARBOHYDRATES: 2g
SUGAR: 1g

Blackened Chicken Tenders

This highly seasoned meal is great if you love a bit of heat. The recipe is named after blackening seasoning, which is spicy and similar to Cajun flavors. For a blackened-style dipping sauce, mix ¼ teaspoon Cajun seasoning in ¼ cup ranch dressing and serve on the side.

- **Pantry Staples: Salt, ground black pepper, paprika, garlic powder, coconut oil**
- **Hands-On Time: 5 minutes**
- **Cook Time: 12 minutes**

Serves 4

1 pound boneless, skinless chicken tenders
2 tablespoons coconut oil, melted
1 teaspoon paprika
½ teaspoon chili powder
½ teaspoon salt
¼ teaspoon ground black pepper
¼ teaspoon garlic powder
¼ teaspoon cayenne pepper

1 In a large bowl, toss chicken tenders in coconut oil. Sprinkle each side of chicken tenders with paprika, chili powder, salt, black pepper, garlic powder, and cayenne pepper.

2 Place tenders into ungreased air fryer basket. Adjust the temperature to 375°F and set the timer for 12 minutes. Tenders will be dark brown and have an internal temperature of at least 165°F when done. Serve warm.

PER SERVING

CALORIES: 156	FAT: 7g
PROTEIN: 21g	SODIUM: 404mg
FIBER: 0g	CARBOHYDRATES: 1g
NET CARBOHYDRATES: 1g	SUGAR: 0g

Butter and Bacon Chicken

This meal is not only easy but also full of flavor. The salty bacon seasons the chicken, so you'll savor every bite. Use leftovers in chicken salad or shredded in taco bowls.

- **Pantry Staples: Salt, ground black pepper, garlic powder**
- **Hands-On Time: 10 minutes**
- **Cook Time: 65 minutes**

Serves 6

1 (4-pound) whole chicken
2 tablespoons salted butter, softened
1 teaspoon dried thyme
½ teaspoon garlic powder
1 teaspoon salt
½ teaspoon ground black pepper
6 slices sugar-free bacon

ROUND OUT THE MEAL!

For a flavorful side, pair this with the Baked Jalapeño and Cheese Cauliflower Mash in Chapter 4. It's the ultimate comfort-food combination—and you never have to turn on your oven!

1 Pat chicken dry with a paper towel, then rub with butter on all sides. Sprinkle thyme, garlic powder, salt, and pepper over chicken.

2 Place chicken into ungreased air fryer basket, breast side up. Lay strips of bacon over chicken and secure with toothpicks.

3 Adjust the temperature to 350°F and set the timer for 65 minutes. Halfway through cooking, remove and set aside bacon and flip chicken over. Chicken will be done when the skin is golden and crispy and the internal temperature is at least 165°F. Serve warm with bacon.

PER SERVING

CALORIES: 416	**FAT:** 26g
PROTEIN: 36g	**SODIUM:** 666mg
FIBER: 0g	**CARBOHYDRATES:** 0g
NET CARBOHYDRATES: 0g	**SUGAR:** 0g

Chicken Cordon Bleu

Traditionally, this recipe calls for breading, but with flavorful ingredients like Dijon mustard and Swiss cheese, you won't even miss it. When buying ham, make sure you choose one that has a "no sugar added" label. Serve with a side of Roasted Broccoli Salad (see recipe in Chapter 4).

- **Pantry Staples: Salt, ground black pepper**
- **Hands-On Time: 15 minutes**
- **Cook Time: 25 minutes**

Serves 4

4 (6-ounce) boneless, skinless chicken breasts

4 (1-ounce) slices Swiss cheese

4 (1-ounce) slices no-sugar-added ham

¼ cup Dijon mustard

½ teaspoon salt

¼ teaspoon ground black pepper

1 Cut a 5"-long slit in the side of each chicken breast. Place a slice of Swiss and a slice of ham inside each slit.

2 Brush chicken with mustard, then sprinkle with salt and pepper on both sides.

3 Place chicken into ungreased air fryer basket. Adjust the temperature to 375°F and set the timer for 25 minutes, turning chicken halfway through cooking. Chicken will be golden brown and have an internal temperature of at least 165°F when done. Serve warm.

PER SERVING

CALORIES: 388	FAT: 14g
PROTEIN: 53g	SODIUM: 1,154mg
FIBER: 0g	CARBOHYDRATES: 3g
NET CARBOHYDRATES: 3g	SUGAR: 0g

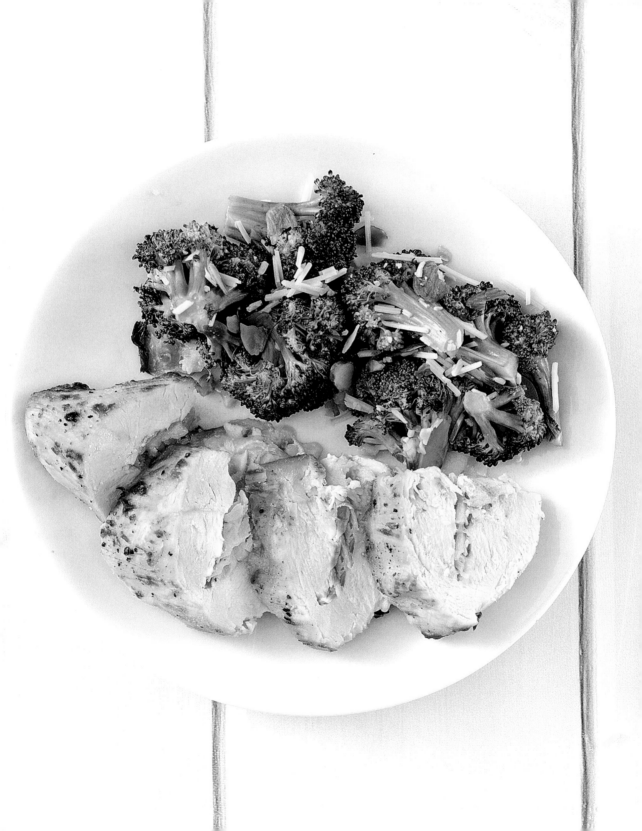

Cheesy Chicken Nuggets

Who can deny the classic flavors of chicken nuggets? They might bring back childhood memories, or they might be your picky kid's favorite thing to eat right now. Either way, this recipe is an irresistible low-carb twist on the traditional breaded nuggets.

- Pantry Staples: Salt, garlic powder
- Hands-On Time: 10 minutes
- Cook Time: 15 minutes

Serves 4

1 pound ground chicken thighs
½ cup shredded mozzarella cheese
1 large egg, whisked
½ teaspoon salt
¼ teaspoon dried oregano
¼ teaspoon garlic powder

1 In a large bowl, combine all ingredients. Form mixture into twenty nugget shapes, about 2 tablespoons each.

2 Place nuggets into ungreased air fryer basket, working in batches if needed. Adjust the temperature to 375°F and set the timer for 15 minutes, turning nuggets halfway through cooking. Let cool 5 minutes before serving.

PER SERVING

CALORIES: 222		FAT: 12g	
PROTEIN: 25g		SODIUM: 472mg	
FIBER: 0g		CARBOHYDRATES: 1g	
NET CARBOHYDRATES: 1g		SUGAR: 0g	

Garlic Ginger Chicken

This recipe is delicious alone, but also makes a great base for a stir-fry. The ginger adds a heat and flavor that go with a variety of vegetables, from mushrooms to cauliflower rice. This recipe uses soy sauce, but feel free to swap for liquid aminos if you prefer.

- **Pantry Staples: Salt**
- **Hands-On Time: 30 minutes**
- **Cook Time: 12 minutes**

Serves 4

1 pound boneless, skinless chicken thighs, cut into 1" pieces

¼ cup soy sauce

2 cloves garlic, peeled and finely minced

1 tablespoon minced ginger

¼ teaspoon salt

1 Place all ingredients in a large sealable bowl or bag. Place sealed bowl or bag into refrigerator and let marinate at least 30 minutes up to overnight.

2 Remove chicken from marinade and place into ungreased air fryer basket. Adjust the temperature to 375°F and set the timer for 12 minutes, shaking the basket twice during cooking. Chicken will be golden and have an internal temperature of at least 165°F when done. Serve warm.

PER SERVING

CALORIES: 140	**FAT:** 6g
PROTEIN: 20g	**SODIUM:** 184mg
FIBER: 0g	**CARBOHYDRATES:** 0g
NET CARBOHYDRATES: 0g	**SUGAR:** 0g

Chipotle Aioli Wings

A major perk of making wings at home is knowing exactly what's going into your batch, so you can avoid the carb-filled seasonings and sauces often used in restaurant options. These wings soak in the flavor of the sauce, and the air fryer cooks them up quickly, so there's no need to marinate in order to get the perfect bite every time.

- **Pantry Staples: Salt, ground black pepper**
- **Hands-On Time: 5 minutes**
- **Cook Time: 25 minutes**

Serves 6

2 pounds bone-in chicken wings
½ teaspoon salt
¼ teaspoon ground black pepper
2 tablespoons mayonnaise
2 teaspoons chipotle powder
2 tablespoons lemon juice

1 In a large bowl, toss wings in salt and pepper, then place into ungreased air fryer basket. Adjust the temperature to 400°F and set the timer for 25 minutes, shaking the basket twice while cooking. Wings will be done when golden and have an internal temperature of at least 165°F.

2 In a small bowl, whisk together mayonnaise, chipotle powder, and lemon juice. Place cooked wings into a large serving bowl and drizzle with aioli. Toss to coat. Serve warm.

PER SERVING

CALORIES: 243
PROTEIN: 19g
FIBER: 0g
NET CARBOHYDRATES: 0g

FAT: 18g
SODIUM: 368mg
CARBOHYDRATES: 0g
SUGAR: 0g

Cajun-Breaded Chicken Bites

Pork rinds make a great alternative to carb-filled panko bread crumbs when you want breading but don't want to cheat on your keto diet. You can easily balance out your fat macros by adding a dipping sauce such as ranch or spicy mayonnaise.

- **Pantry Staples:** Salt, ground black pepper
- **Hands-On Time:** 10 minutes
- **Cook Time:** 12 minutes

Serves 4

1 pound boneless, skinless chicken breasts, cut into 1" cubes

½ cup heavy whipping cream

½ teaspoon salt

¼ teaspoon ground black pepper

1 ounce plain pork rinds, finely crushed

¼ cup unflavored whey protein powder

½ teaspoon Cajun seasoning

1 Place chicken in a medium bowl and pour in cream. Stir to coat. Sprinkle with salt and pepper.

2 In a separate large bowl, combine pork rinds, protein powder, and Cajun seasoning. Remove chicken from cream, shaking off any excess, and toss in dry mix until fully coated.

3 Place bites into ungreased air fryer basket. Adjust the temperature to 400°F and set the timer for 12 minutes, shaking the basket twice during cooking. Bites will be done when golden brown and have an internal temperature of at least 165°F. Serve warm.

PER SERVING

CALORIES: 285

PROTEIN: 34g

FIBER: 0g

NET CARBOHYDRATES: 1g

FAT: 16g

SODIUM: 497mg

CARBOHYDRATES: 1g

SUGAR: 1g

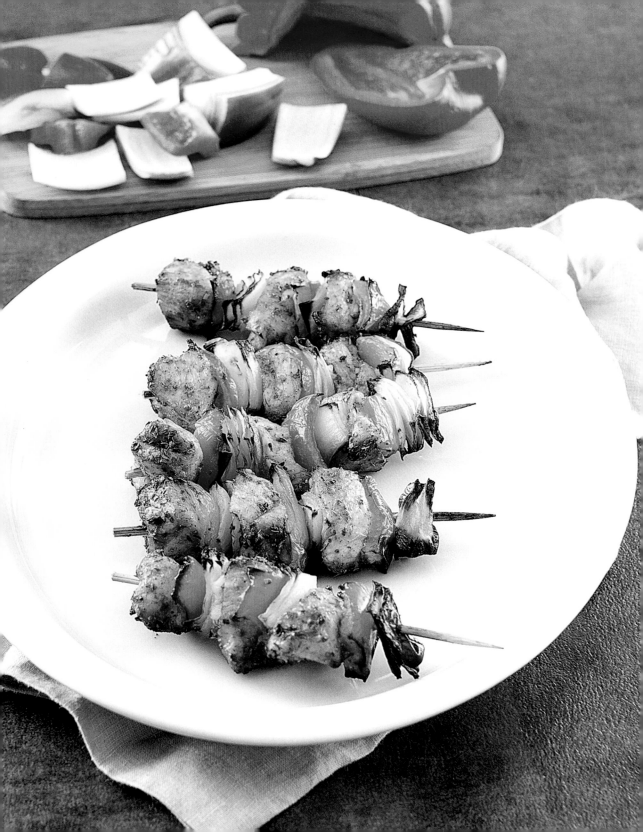

Jerk Chicken Kebabs

Air fryer kebabs are delicious and packed with flavor. T?
melized, giving vegetables a sweeter roasted taste. Yo?
toss the cooked ingredients into a salad or serve over

- **Pantry Staples: Salt, coconut oil**
- **Hands-On Time: 10 minutes**
- **Cook Time: 14 minutes**

Serves 4

8 ounces boneless, skinless chicken thighs, cut into 1" cubes

2 tablespoons jerk seasoning

2 tablespoons coconut oil

½ medium red bell pepper, seeded and cut into 1" pieces

¼ medium red onion, peeled and cut into 1" pieces

½ teaspoon salt

HIDDEN SUGAR

Always make sure to read your labels. Jerk seasoning is naturally very spicy, so it's common to see sugar added to commercial brands to offset the heat. Look for blends that don't have added sugar.

1 Place chick?
   with jerk s?
   coat on al?

2 Using eight 6" skewers, bui??
   alternating chicken, pepper, and onion pieces, about three repetitions per skewer.

3 Sprinkle salt over skewers and place into ungreased air fryer basket. Adjust the temperature to 370°F and set the timer for 14 minutes, turning skewers halfway through cooking. Chicken will be golden and have an internal temperature of at least 165°F when done. Serve warm.

PER SERVING

CALORIES: 138	**FAT:** 7g
PROTEIN: 10g	**SODIUM:** 550mg
FIBER: 0g	**CARBOHYDRATES:** 2g
NET CARBOHYDRATES: 2g	**SUGAR:** 1g

Turmeric Chicken Thighs

...ginger are two anti-inflammatory spices that can boost immunity and ...th. As an added bonus, they're both bursting with savory flavors that perfectly ...ent a fatty cut of meat like chicken thigh. Toss leftovers into a chicken salad for a ...classic greens.

- **Pantry Staples: Salt, ground black pepper, garlic powder, coconut oil**
- **Hands-On Time: 5 minutes**
- **Cook Time: 25 minutes**

Serves 4

4 (4-ounce) boneless, skin-on chicken thighs

2 tablespoons coconut oil, melted

½ teaspoon ground turmeric

½ teaspoon salt

½ teaspoon garlic powder

½ teaspoon ground ginger

¼ teaspoon ground black pepper

1 Place chicken thighs in a large bowl and drizzle with coconut oil. Sprinkle with remaining ingredients and toss to coat both sides of thighs.

2 Place thighs skin side up into ungreased air fryer basket. Adjust the temperature to 400°F and set the timer for 25 minutes. After 10 minutes, turn thighs. When 5 minutes remain, flip thighs once more. Chicken will be done when skin is golden brown and the internal temperature is at least 165°F. Serve warm.

PER SERVING

CALORIES: 306	FAT: 17g
PROTEIN: 34g	SODIUM: 435mg
FIBER: 0g	CARBOHYDRATES: 1g
NET CARBOHYDRATES: 1g	SUGAR: 0g

Tangy Mustard Wings

If you're a fan of salt and vinegar flavor, this recipe is a must try! These wings are tangy without tasting overly like mustard. They are so bursting with flavor, you won't even need a dipping sauce.

- **Pantry Staples: Salt, ground black pepper**
- **Hands-On Time: 5 minutes**
- **Cook Time: 25 minutes**

Serves 4

1 pound bone-in chicken wings, separated at joints
¼ cup yellow mustard
½ teaspoon salt
¼ teaspoon ground black pepper

1 Place wings in a large bowl and toss with mustard to fully coat. Sprinkle with salt and pepper.

2 Place wings into ungreased air fryer basket. Adjust the temperature to 400°F and set the timer for 25 minutes, shaking the basket three times during cooking. Wings will be done when browned and cooked to an internal temperature of at least 165°F. Serve warm.

PER SERVING

CALORIES: 182	FAT: 12g
PROTEIN: 16g	SODIUM: 538mg
FIBER: 1g	CARBOHYDRATES: 1g
NET CARBOHYDRATES: 0g	SUGAR: 0g

Hasselback Alfredo Chicken

Alfredo sauce is naturally low in carbs and high in fat, which makes it perfect for the keto diet. This recipe uses the creamy flavor of Alfredo in every bite, making it a soon-to-be weeknight favorite. Feel free to leave out the pepper flakes if you prefer less heat.

- Pantry Staples: Salt, ground black pepper, coconut oil
- Hands-On Time: 10 minutes
- Cook Time: 20 minutes

Serves 4

4 (6-ounce) boneless, skinless chicken breasts
4 teaspoons coconut oil
½ teaspoon salt
¼ teaspoon ground black pepper
4 strips cooked sugar-free bacon, broken into 24 pieces
½ cup Alfredo sauce
1 cup shredded mozzarella cheese
¼ teaspoon crushed red pepper flakes

1 Cut six horizontal slits in the top of each chicken breast. Drizzle with coconut oil and sprinkle with salt and black pepper. Place into an ungreased 6″ round nonstick baking dish.

2 Place 1 bacon piece in each slit in chicken breasts. Pour Alfredo sauce over chicken and sprinkle with mozzarella and red pepper flakes.

3 Place dish into air fryer basket. Adjust the temperature to 370°F and set the timer for 20 minutes. Chicken will be done when internal temperature is at least 165°F and cheese is browned. Serve warm.

PER SERVING

CALORIES: 396
PROTEIN: 49g
FIBER: 0g
NET CARBOHYDRATES: 3g

FAT: 17g
SODIUM: 921mg
CARBOHYDRATES: 3g
SUGAR: 1g

Jumbo Buffalo Chicken Meatballs

These spicy meatballs are bursting with flavor. They're perfect for anyone who loves the classic combination of buffalo sauce and blue cheese. They are also great for meal prep and can be frozen after cooking. Enjoy with celery sticks and ranch for dipping.

- **Pantry Staples: Salt, ground black pepper**
- **Hands-On Time: 5 minutes**
- **Cook Time: 15 minutes**

Serves 4

1 pound ground chicken thighs

1 large egg, whisked

½ cup hot sauce, divided

½ cup crumbled blue cheese

2 tablespoons dry ranch seasoning

¼ teaspoon salt

¼ teaspoon ground black pepper

FREEZER-FRIENDLY MEATBALLS

To freeze these meatballs after cooking, simply place them on a medium ungreased parchment-lined baking tray and put in the freezer for 1 hour. Then place the frozen meatballs in a sealable freezer bag for up to 3 months.

1 In a large bowl, combine ground chicken, egg, ¼ cup hot sauce, blue cheese, ranch seasoning, salt, and pepper.

2 Divide mixture into eight equal sections of about ¼ cup each and form each section into a ball. Place meatballs into ungreased air fryer basket. Adjust the temperature to 370°F and set the timer for 15 minutes. Meatballs will be done when golden and have an internal temperature of at least 165°F.

3 Transfer meatballs to a large serving dish and toss with remaining hot sauce. Serve warm.

PER SERVING

CALORIES: 254	FAT: 14g
PROTEIN: 25g	SODIUM: 1,749mg
FIBER: 0g	CARBOHYDRATES: 4g
NET CARBOHYDRATES: 4g	SUGAR: 0g

6

Beef and Pork Main Dishes

Beef and pork are great for any low-carb diet such as keto, but sometimes it can be difficult to know what to do with them, especially when you're short on time and ingredients. The air fryer is a quick and easy way to take your beef and pork dishes to the next level.

Say goodbye to boring meats and long lists of overly complicated ingredients thanks to the perfectly seasoned, fast-cooking range of recipes in this chapter! In practically no time at all—and with just five ingredients or less—you'll be serving everything from juicy Sweet and Spicy Spare Ribs and Pork Meatballs to delicious Marinated Rib Eye and London Broil.

Mozzarella-Stuffed Meatloaf

There's nothing plain or boring about this meatloaf! Filled with nutritious vegetables and gooey cheese, it's a dish you can feel great about serving your family. Plus, with the air fryer's quick cooking time, you'll have dinner on the table in no time!

- **Pantry Staples: Salt, ground black pepper**
- **Hands-On Time: 10 minutes**
- **Cook Time: 30 minutes**

Serves 6

1 pound 80/20 ground beef

½ medium green bell pepper, seeded and chopped

¼ medium yellow onion, peeled and chopped

½ teaspoon salt

¼ teaspoon ground black pepper

2 ounces mozzarella cheese, sliced into ¼"-thick slices

¼ cup low-carb ketchup

1 In a large bowl, combine ground beef, bell pepper, onion, salt, and black pepper. Cut a piece of parchment to fit air fryer basket. Place half beef mixture on ungreased parchment and form a 9″ × 4″ loaf, about ½″ thick.

2 Center mozzarella slices on beef loaf, leaving at least ¼″ around each edge.

3 Press remaining beef into a second 9″ × 4″ loaf and place on top of mozzarella, pressing edges of loaves together to seal.

4 Place parchment with meatloaf into air fryer basket. Adjust the temperature to 350°F and set the timer for 30 minutes, carefully turning loaf and brushing top with ketchup halfway through cooking. Loaf will be browned and have an internal temperature of at least 180°F when done. Slice and serve warm.

PER SERVING

CALORIES: 227

PROTEIN: 15g

FIBER: 0g

NET CARBOHYDRATES: 2g

FAT: 14g

SODIUM: 434mg

CARBOHYDRATES: 2g

SUGAR: 1g

Marinated Steak Kebabs

Beef kebabs are a great, well-rounded dinner for any night of the week. And there's no need to fire up the grill for this delicious recipe! The meat should be marinated for at least 30 minutes before cooking, but it can marinate for up to 24 hours in the refrigerator if you're preparing this meal the night before.

- **Pantry Staples: Salt, ground black pepper**
- **Hands-On Time: 45 minutes**
- **Cook Time: 5 minutes**

Serves 4

1 pound strip steak, fat trimmed, cut into 1" cubes
½ cup soy sauce
¼ cup olive oil
1 tablespoon granular brown erythritol
½ teaspoon salt
¼ teaspoon ground black pepper
1 medium green bell pepper, seeded and chopped into 1" cubes

1   Place steak into a large sealable bowl or bag and pour in soy sauce and olive oil. Add erythritol, then stir to coat steak. Marinate at room temperature 30 minutes.

2   Remove streak from marinade and sprinkle with salt and black pepper.

3   Place meat and vegetables onto 6" skewer sticks, alternating between steak and bell pepper.

4   Place kebabs into ungreased air fryer basket. Adjust the temperature to 400°F and set the timer for 5 minutes. Steak will be done when crispy at the edges and peppers are tender. Serve warm.

PER SERVING

CALORIES: 277	FAT: 17g
PROTEIN: 24g	SODIUM: 525mg
FIBER: 1g	CARBOHYDRATES: 2g
NET CARBOHYDRATES: 1g	SUGAR: 1g

Cheese-Stuffed Steak Burgers

This recipe takes your burger game to the next level. Instead of ground beef, it uses flavorful sirloin stuffed with gooey cheese. Make this your own by swapping out the Cheddar cheese for pepper jack or American.

- **Pantry Staples: Salt, ground black pepper**
- **Hands-On Time: 10 minutes**
- **Cook Time: 10 minutes**

Serves 4

1 pound 80/20 ground sirloin

4 ounces mild Cheddar cheese, cubed

½ teaspoon salt

¼ teaspoon ground black pepper

1 Form ground sirloin into four equal balls, then separate each ball in half and flatten into two thin patties, for eight total patties. Place 1 ounce Cheddar into center of one patty, then top with a second patty and press edges to seal burger closed. Repeat with remaining patties and Cheddar to create four burgers.

2 Sprinkle salt and pepper over both sides of burgers and carefully place burgers into ungreased air fryer basket. Adjust the temperature to 350°F and set the timer for 10 minutes. Burgers will be done when browned on the edges and top. Serve warm.

PER SERVING

CALORIES: 323
PROTEIN: 27g
FIBER: 0g
NET CARBOHYDRATES: 0g

FAT: 20g
SODIUM: 530mg
CARBOHYDRATES: 0g
SUGAR: 0g

Corn Dogs

This recipe is a keto-friendly alternative to the traditional carb-loaded version. Typically, corn dogs are coated in cornmeal, but this recipe gives them a low-carb, cheesy twist. Serve with your favorite mustard or low-carb ketchup for dipping.

- **Pantry Staples: None**
- **Hands-On Time: 10 minutes**
- **Cook Time: 8 minutes**

Serves 4

1½ cups shredded mozzarella cheese

1 ounce cream cheese

½ cup blanched finely ground almond flour

4 beef hot dogs

THE FEWER INGREDIENTS, THE BETTER

Opt for higher-quality hot dogs and sausages with only a few ingredients on the label. Many of the value varieties are combinations of low-quality chicken, pork, and beef, along with unhealthy preservatives and high-fructose corn syrup. All-beef hot dogs with no nitrates are a healthier, keto-friendly choice.

1   Place mozzarella, cream cheese, and flour in a large microwave-safe bowl. Microwave on high 45 seconds, then stir with a fork until a soft ball of dough forms.

2   Press dough out into a 12″ × 6″ rectangle, then use a knife to separate into four smaller rectangles.

3   Wrap each hot dog in one rectangle of dough and place into ungreased air fryer basket. Adjust the temperature to 400°F and set the timer for 8 minutes, turning corn dogs halfway through cooking. Corn dogs will be golden brown when done. Serve warm.

PER SERVING

CALORIES: 348

PROTEIN: 18g

FIBER: 1g

NET CARBOHYDRATES: 5g

FAT: 25g

SODIUM: 723mg

CARBOHYDRATES: 6g

SUGAR: 2g

Mustard Herb Pork Tenderloin

This recipe is perfect for family dinners. It's easy to prep, but your guests would never know it! The mustard does the work for you, providing a smooth and slightly sweet base for the herb crust. Pair with the Dinner Rolls in Chapter 4 for a comforting family meal.

- **Pantry Staples: Salt, ground black pepper**
- **Hands-On Time: 5 minutes**
- **Cook Time: 20 minutes**

Serves 6

¼ cup mayonnaise

2 tablespoons Dijon mustard

½ teaspoon dried thyme

¼ teaspoon dried rosemary

1 (1-pound) pork tenderloin

½ teaspoon salt

¼ teaspoon ground black pepper

1 In a small bowl, mix mayonnaise, mustard, thyme, and rosemary. Brush tenderloin with mixture on all sides, then sprinkle with salt and pepper on all sides.

2 Place tenderloin into ungreased air fryer basket. Adjust the temperature to 400°F and set the timer for 20 minutes, turning tenderloin halfway through cooking. Tenderloin will be golden and have an internal temperature of at least 145°F when done. Serve warm.

PER SERVING

CALORIES: 158

PROTEIN: 16g

FIBER: 0g

NET CARBOHYDRATES: 1g

FAT: 9g

SODIUM: 557mg

CARBOHYDRATES: 1g

SUGAR: 0g

Bacon-Wrapped Pork Tenderloin

The best part about this dish is that there's bacon in every bite! Pork can easily dry out under high heat, so adding the fat from the bacon locks in all the deliciousness for a low-cost meal that's packed with flavor. Serve with a side of Parmesan Herb Radishes (see recipe in Chapter 4).

- **Pantry Staples: Salt, ground black pepper, garlic powder**
- **Hands-On Time: 10 minutes**
- **Cook Time: 20 minutes**

Serves 6

1 (1-pound) pork tenderloin
½ teaspoon salt
½ teaspoon garlic powder
¼ teaspoon ground black pepper
8 slices sugar-free bacon

1 Sprinkle tenderloin with salt, garlic powder, and pepper. Wrap each piece of bacon around tenderloin and secure with toothpicks.

2 Place tenderloin into ungreased air fryer basket. Adjust the temperature to 400°F and set the timer for 20 minutes, turning tenderloin after 15 minutes. When done, bacon will be crispy and tenderloin will have an internal temperature of at least 145°F.

3 Cut the tenderloin into six even portions and transfer each to a medium plate and serve warm.

PER SERVING

CALORIES: 144
PROTEIN: 20g
FIBER: 0g
NET CARBOHYDRATES: 0g

FAT: 6g
SODIUM: 590mg
CARBOHYDRATES: 0g
SUGAR: 0g

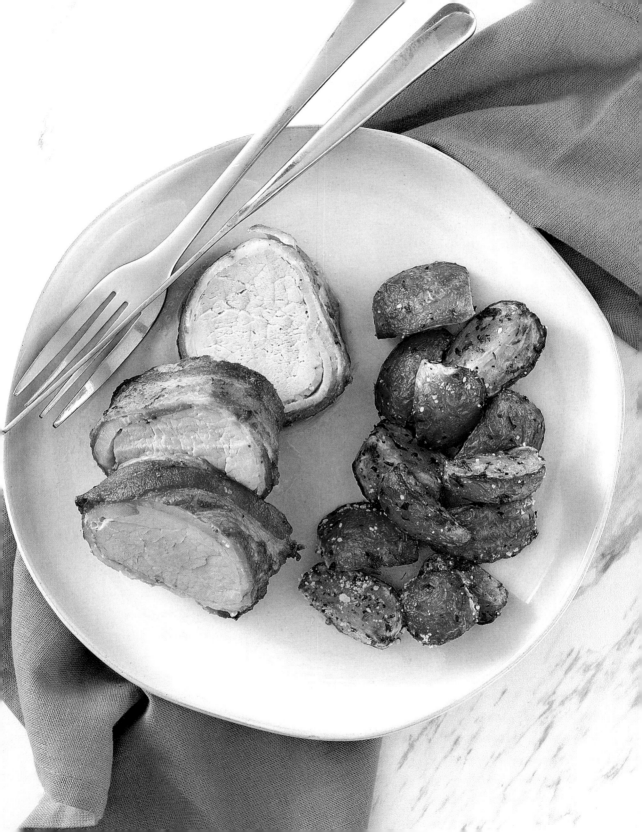

Buttery Pork Chops

You'll be amazed how perfectly air fryers cook pork chops. A dark-golden crust forms on each side, leaving the inside tender and moist. Adding your favorite seasonings can spice things up, but these are delicious and melt in your mouth with just salt and pepper.

- **Pantry Staples: Salt, ground black pepper**
- **Hands-On Time: 5 minutes**
- **Cook Time: 12 minutes**

Serves 4

4 (4-ounce) boneless pork chops

½ teaspoon salt

¼ teaspoon ground black pepper

2 tablespoons salted butter, softened

1 Sprinkle pork chops on all sides with salt and pepper. Place chops into ungreased air fryer basket in a single layer. Adjust the temperature to 400°F and set the timer for 12 minutes. Pork chops will be golden and have an internal temperature of at least 145°F when done.

2 Use tongs to remove cooked pork chops from air fryer and place onto a large plate. Top each chop with ½ tablespoon butter and let sit 2 minutes to melt. Serve warm.

PER SERVING

CALORIES: 278
PROTEIN: 24g
FIBER: 0g
NET CARBOHYDRATES: 0g

FAT: 19g
SODIUM: 428mg
CARBOHYDRATES: 0g
SUGAR: 0g

Bacon and Cheese–Stuffed Pork Chops

Pork chops are a great budget meal but don't always get the attention they deserve. This delicious recipe stuffs them with salty bacon and cheese for amazing flavor in every bite. It's a meal the whole family can enjoy.

- **Pantry Staples: Salt, ground black pepper**
- **Hands-On Time: 10 minutes**
- **Cook Time: 12 minutes**

Serves 4

½ ounce plain pork rinds, finely crushed

½ cup shredded sharp Cheddar cheese

4 slices cooked sugar-free bacon, crumbled

4 (4-ounce) boneless pork chops

½ teaspoon salt

¼ teaspoon ground black pepper

1 In a small bowl, mix pork rinds, Cheddar, and bacon.

2 Make a 3″ slit in the side of each pork chop and stuff with ¼ pork rind mixture. Sprinkle each side of pork chops with salt and pepper.

3 Place pork chops into ungreased air fryer basket, stuffed side up. Adjust the temperature to 400°F and set the timer for 12 minutes. Pork chops will be browned and have an internal temperature of at least 145°F when done. Serve warm.

PER SERVING

CALORIES: 348
PROTEIN: 33g
FIBER: 0g
NET CARBOHYDRATES: 0g

FAT: 22g
SODIUM: 694mg
CARBOHYDRATES: 0g
SUGAR: 0g

GIVE THEM A PERSONAL TOUCH!

Make this recipe your own by adding your favorite seasonings to the outside of the pork before baking. You can add an herb blend, Cajun seasoning, or barbecue dry rub—you may even find an unexpected combination that you love!

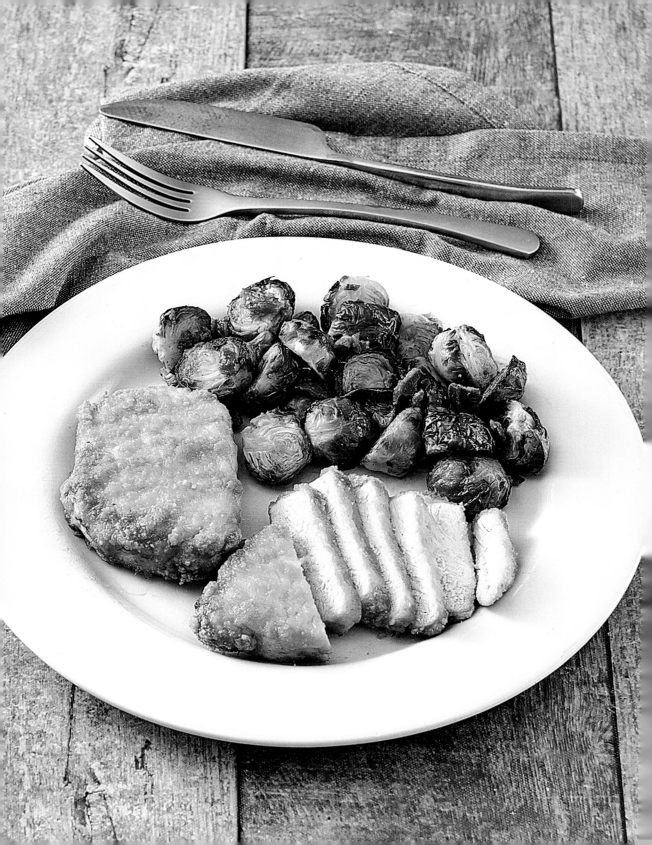

Parmesan-Crusted Pork Chops

While you may not typically think of cheese and pork together, this recipe may change your mind. A delicious thick crust forms on the cheese and gives the juicy pork even more flavor. Add a teaspoon of Italian seasoning for an extra kick. Round out the meal with a side of Bacon-Balsamic Brussels Sprouts (see recipe in Chapter 4).

- **Pantry Staples: Salt, ground black pepper**
- **Hands-On Time: 5 minutes**
- **Cook Time: 12 minutes**

Serves 4

1 large egg

½ cup grated Parmesan cheese

4 (4-ounce) boneless pork chops

½ teaspoon salt

¼ teaspoon ground black pepper

1 Whisk egg in a medium bowl and place Parmesan in a separate medium bowl.

2 Sprinkle pork chops on both sides with salt and pepper. Dip each pork chop into egg, then press both sides into Parmesan.

3 Place pork chops into ungreased air fryer basket. Adjust the temperature to 400°F and set the timer for 12 minutes, turning chops halfway through cooking. Pork chops will be golden and have an internal temperature of at least 145°F when done. Serve warm.

PER SERVING

CALORIES: 298	**FAT:** 17g
PROTEIN: 29g	**SODIUM:** 626mg
FIBER: 0g	**CARBOHYDRATES:** 2g
NET CARBOHYDRATES: 2g	**SUGAR:** 0g

Marinated Rib Eye

Yes, you can achieve perfectly cooked rib eye using only your air fryer! It's a great time-saver, as opposed to the skillet or grill, and the flavor is just as delicious. The quick marinade in this recipe takes things to the next level—the keto-friendly erythritol gives it just a hint of sweetness.

- **Pantry Staples: Salt, ground black pepper**
- **Hands-On Time: 35 minutes**
- **Cook Time: 10 minutes**

Serves 4

1 pound rib eye steak

¼ cup soy sauce

1 tablespoon Worcestershire sauce

1 tablespoon granular brown erythritol

2 tablespoons olive oil

½ teaspoon salt

¼ teaspoon ground black pepper

1 Place rib eye in a large sealable bowl or bag and pour in soy sauce, Worcestershire sauce, erythritol, and olive oil. Seal and let marinate 30 minutes in the refrigerator.

2 Remove rib eye from marinade, pat dry, and sprinkle on all sides with salt and pepper. Place rib eye into ungreased air fryer basket. Adjust the temperature to 400°F and set the timer for 10 minutes. Steak will be done when browned at the edges and has an internal temperature of 150°F for medium or 180°F for well-done. Serve warm.

PER SERVING

CALORIES: 350	FAT: 26g
PROTEIN: 26g	SODIUM: 443mg
FIBER: 0g	CARBOHYDRATES: 1g
NET CARBOHYDRATES: 1g	SUGAR: 0g

MARINATING MEATS

Marinating adds flavor and helps to tenderize tougher cuts of meat. Most meats should be marinated for at least 30 minutes, but you can choose to let them marinate overnight in the refrigerator to soak up as much flavor as possible. Just remember to pat the meat dry before placing it into the air fryer.

Crispy Pork Belly

Pork belly is cut from the same area as bacon but is uncured and often sliced in larger chunks. Think of it as a big slab of bacon that you can crisp up and eat like a popper. You can make this a meal or even a superfilling snack—just be sure to plan ahead so the meat has time to marinate.

- **Pantry Staples: Salt, ground black pepper**
- **Hands-On Time: 40 minutes**
- **Cook Time: 20 minutes**

Serves 4

1 pound pork belly, cut into 1" cubes

¼ cup soy sauce

1 tablespoon Worcestershire sauce

2 teaspoons sriracha hot chili sauce

½ teaspoon salt

¼ teaspoon ground black pepper

WHERE TO FIND PORK BELLY

Typically, you can find pork belly in the meat section of the grocery store. You may need to ask for it from the butcher. If you have trouble finding it, try a natural grocery store. They may also have a fresher selection of meat.

1 Place pork belly into a medium sealable bowl or bag and pour in soy sauce, Worcestershire sauce, and sriracha. Seal and let marinate 30 minutes in the refrigerator.

2 Remove pork from marinade, pat dry with a paper towel, and sprinkle with salt and pepper.

3 Place pork in ungreased air fryer basket. Adjust the temperature to 360°F and set the timer for 20 minutes, shaking the basket halfway through cooking. Pork belly will be done when it has an internal temperature of at least 145°F and is golden brown.

4 Let pork belly rest on a large plate 10 minutes. Serve warm.

PER SERVING

CALORIES: 588	FAT: 56g
PROTEIN: 11g	SODIUM: 423mg
FIBER: 0g	CARBOHYDRATES: 0g
NET CARBOHYDRATES: 0g	SUGAR: 0g

Pork Spare Ribs

Cooking tender, juicy ribs has never been easier, thanks to the air fryer. The sauce in this recipe caramelizes to create a thick glaze that makes the perfect bite. Pair with cauliflower rice for a filling family dinner.

- **Pantry Staples: Salt, ground black pepper, garlic powder**
- **Hands-On Time: 10 minutes**
- **Cook Time: 30 minutes**

Serves 4

1 (4-pound) rack pork spare ribs

1 teaspoon ground cumin

2 teaspoons salt

1 teaspoon ground black pepper

1 teaspoon garlic powder

½ teaspoon dry ground mustard

½ cup low-carb barbecue sauce

1. Place ribs on ungreased aluminum foil sheet. Carefully use a knife to remove membrane and sprinkle meat evenly on both sides with cumin, salt, pepper, garlic powder, and ground mustard.

2. Cut rack into portions that will fit in your air fryer, and wrap each portion in one layer of aluminum foil, working in batches if needed.

3. Place ribs into ungreased air fryer basket. Adjust the temperature to 400°F and set the timer for 25 minutes.

4. When the timer beeps, carefully remove ribs from foil and brush with barbecue sauce. Return to air fryer and cook at 400°F for an additional 5 minutes to brown. Ribs will be done when no pink remains and internal temperature is at least 180°F. Serve warm.

PER SERVING

CALORIES: 192	**FAT:** 12g
PROTEIN: 13g	**SODIUM:** 1,374mg
FIBER: 0g	**CARBOHYDRATES:** 3g
NET CARBOHYDRATES: 3g	**SUGAR:** 0g

Sweet and Spicy Spare Ribs

These ribs are packed with so much flavor that you won't even miss the barbecue sauce. The first thing you'll taste is the sweetness, then you'll get a mild heat that slowly builds and leaves you wanting more.

- **Pantry Staples: Salt, ground black pepper, paprika, garlic powder**
- **Hands-On Time: 10 minutes**
- **Cook Time: 30 minutes**

Serves 6

¼ cup granular brown erythritol

2 teaspoons paprika

2 teaspoons chili powder

1 teaspoon garlic powder

½ teaspoon cayenne pepper

2 teaspoons salt

1 teaspoon ground black pepper

1 (4-pound) rack pork spare ribs

1. In a small bowl, mix erythritol, paprika, chili powder, garlic powder, cayenne pepper, salt, and black pepper. Rub spice mix over ribs on both sides. Place ribs on ungreased aluminum foil sheet and wrap to cover.

2. Place ribs into ungreased air fryer basket. Adjust the temperature to 400°F and set the timer for 25 minutes.

3. When timer beeps, remove ribs from foil, then place back into air fryer basket to cook an additional 5 minutes, turning halfway through cooking. Ribs will be browned and have an internal temperature of at least 180°F when done. Serve warm.

PER SERVING

CALORIES: 474	FAT: 32g
PROTEIN: 35g	SODIUM: 898mg
FIBER: 1g	CARBOHYDRATES: 9g
NET CARBOHYDRATES: 0g	SUGAR: 0g
SUGAR ALCOHOL: 8g	

Italian Meatballs

Baked meatballs are always delicious, but in the air fryer they cook in less time and don't require heating up an oven. These herb-filled meatballs are the perfect companion for zucchini noodles and low-carb marinara.

- **Pantry Staples: Salt, ground black pepper**
- **Hands-On Time: 10 minutes**
- **Cook Time: 20 minutes**

Serves 4

1 pound 80/20 ground beef

1 large egg, whisked

¼ cup grated Parmesan cheese

½ teaspoon salt

½ teaspoon dried parsley

¼ teaspoon ground black pepper

¼ teaspoon dried oregano

1. In a large bowl, combine all ingredients. Scoop out 3 tablespoons mixture and roll into a ball. Repeat with remaining mixture to form sixteen balls total.

2. Place meatballs into ungreased air fryer basket in a single layer, working in batches if needed. Adjust the temperature to 400°F and set the timer for 20 minutes, shaking the basket halfway through cooking. Meatballs will be browned and have an internal temperature of at least 180°F when done. Serve warm.

PER SERVING

CALORIES: 234	FAT: 13g
PROTEIN: 23g	SODIUM: 382mg
FIBER: 0g	CARBOHYDRATES: 0g
NET CARBOHYDRATES: 0g	SUGAR: 0g

LOVE YOUR LEFTOVERS!

Turn leftovers into a flavorful casserole. Place meatballs into a 6″ round nonstick baking dish and top with dollops of herb-seasoned ricotta cheese. Pour ½ cup low-carb marinara over meatballs and ricotta, and sprinkle with ½ cup shredded mozzarella cheese. Bake in the air fryer at 350°F for 15 minutes.

Roast Beef

The classic comfort food just got even easier in the air fryer! A dark, crispy layer forms on the outside of the meat and locks in flavor, leaving the roast juicy inside. For a complete meal, add chopped vegetables around the roast during the last 15 minutes of cooking.

- **Pantry Staples: Salt, ground black pepper, garlic powder, coconut oil**
- **Hands-On Time: 5 minutes**
- **Cook Time: 60 minutes**

Serves 6

1 (2-pound) top round beef roast
1 teaspoon salt
½ teaspoon ground black pepper
1 teaspoon dried rosemary
½ teaspoon garlic powder
1 tablespoon coconut oil, melted

Sprinkle all sides of roast with salt, pepper, rosemary, and garlic powder. Drizzle with coconut oil. Place roast into ungreased air fryer basket, fatty side down. Adjust the temperature to 375°F and set the timer for 60 minutes, turning the roast halfway through cooking. Roast will be done when no pink remains and internal temperature is at least 180°F. Serve warm.

PER SERVING

CALORIES: 184	FAT: 5g
PROTEIN: 33g	SODIUM: 460mg
FIBER: 0g	CARBOHYDRATES: 0g
NET CARBOHYDRATES: 0g	SUGAR: 0g

Mexican-Style Shredded Beef

This recipe has a deep flavor that makes it great for a variety of meals. The quick prep time also makes it a good option when you're running low on time. Serve it over buttery cauliflower rice and top with sour cream, guacamole, and cheese for a filling taco bowl.

- **Pantry Staples: Salt, ground black pepper**
- **Hands-On Time: 5 minutes**
- **Cook Time: 35 minutes**

Serves 6

1 (2-pound) beef chuck roast, cut into 2" cubes
1 teaspoon salt
½ teaspoon ground black pepper
½ cup no-sugar-added chipotle sauce

1 In a large bowl, sprinkle beef cubes with salt and pepper and toss to coat. Place beef into ungreased air fryer basket. Adjust the temperature to 400°F and set the timer for 30 minutes, shaking the basket halfway through cooking. Beef will be done when internal temperature is at least 160°F.

2 Place cooked beef into a large bowl and shred with two forks. Pour in chipotle sauce and toss to coat.

3 Return beef to air fryer basket for an additional 5 minutes at 400°F to crisp with sauce. Serve warm.

PER SERVING

CALORIES: 217	FAT: 6g
PROTEIN: 37g	SODIUM: 807mg
FIBER: 0g	CARBOHYDRATES: 0g
NET CARBOHYDRATES: 0g	SUGAR: 0g

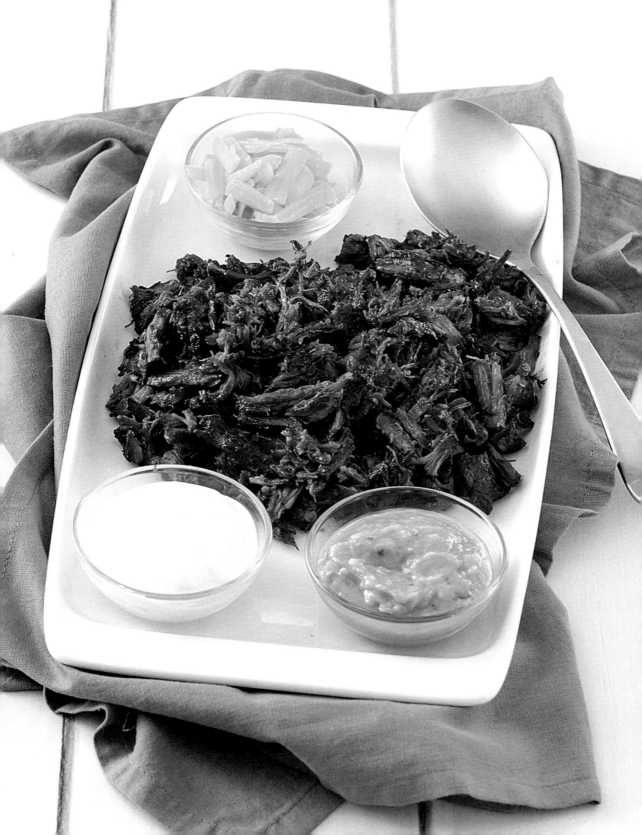

Pork Meatballs

This dish is inspired by the flavors of the classic egg roll. Ground pork tends to be lean, so be sure to pair this recipe with a side that is higher in fat to balance out the meal.

- **Pantry Staples: Salt, garlic powder**
- **Hands-On Time: 10 minutes**
- **Cook Time: 12 minutes**

Yields 18 meatballs

1 pound ground pork
1 large egg, whisked
½ teaspoon garlic powder
½ teaspoon salt
½ teaspoon ground ginger
¼ teaspoon crushed red pepper flakes
1 medium scallion, trimmed and sliced

LOW-FAT MEAT ON THE KETO DIET

On a ketogenic diet, your overall macros will be higher in fat, but this doesn't mean that you need to eat only fatty cuts of meat. Just make sure you're hitting your protein goal and then enjoy fats within your daily range as needed.

1. Combine all ingredients in a large bowl. Spoon out 2 tablespoons mixture and roll into a ball. Repeat to form eighteen meatballs total.

2. Place meatballs into ungreased air fryer basket. Adjust the temperature to 400°F and set the timer for 12 minutes, shaking the basket three times throughout cooking. Meatballs will be browned and have an internal temperature of at least 145°F when done. Serve warm.

PER SERVING (3 MEATBALLS)

CALORIES: 164	**FAT:** 10g
PROTEIN: 15g	**SODIUM:** 252mg
FIBER: 0g	**CARBOHYDRATES:** 1g
NET CARBOHYDRATES: 1g	**SUGAR:** 0g

London Broil

This is the perfect weekend dinner. Just because you may have extra time to cook doesn't mean you want to spend that time in the kitchen. Whip up this London Broil in no time with just a few ingredients!

- **Pantry Staples: Salt, ground black pepper**
- **Hands-On Time: 2 hours**
- **Cook Time: 12 minutes**

Serves 4

1 pound top round steak

1 tablespoon Worcestershire sauce

¼ cup soy sauce

2 cloves garlic, peeled and finely minced

½ teaspoon ground black pepper

½ teaspoon salt

2 tablespoons salted butter, melted

1 Place steak in a large sealable bowl or bag. Pour in Worcestershire sauce and soy sauce, then add garlic, pepper, and salt. Toss to coat. Seal and place into refrigerator to let marinate 2 hours.

2 Remove steak from marinade and pat dry. Drizzle top side with butter, then place into ungreased air fryer basket. Adjust the temperature to 375°F and set the timer for 12 minutes, turning steak halfway through cooking. Steak will be done when browned at the edges and it has an internal temperature of 150°F for medium or 180°F for well-done.

3 Let steak rest on a large plate 10 minutes before slicing into thin pieces. Serve warm.

PER SERVING

CALORIES: 174
PROTEIN: 25g
FIBER: 0g
NET CARBOHYDRATES: 0g

FAT: 8g
SODIUM: 220mg
CARBOHYDRATES: 0g
SUGAR: 0g

Spice-Rubbed Pork Loin

The best things about pork are that it's inexpensive and has a mild flavor that makes it the perfect blank canvas for your seasoning. Pair this dish with Roasted Brussels Sprouts (see recipe in Chapter 4) for a complete meal that can be done in just over 20 minutes!

- **Pantry Staples: Salt, ground black pepper, paprika, garlic powder, coconut oil**
- **Hands-On Time: 5 minutes**
- **Cook Time: 20 minutes**

Serves 6

1 teaspoon paprika
½ teaspoon ground cumin
½ teaspoon chili powder
½ teaspoon garlic powder
2 tablespoons coconut oil
1 (1½-pound) boneless pork loin
½ teaspoon salt
¼ teaspoon ground black pepper

1 In a small bowl, mix paprika, cumin, chili powder, and garlic powder.

2 Drizzle coconut oil over pork. Sprinkle pork loin with salt and pepper, then rub spice mixture evenly on all sides.

3 Place pork loin into ungreased air fryer basket. Adjust the temperature to 400°F and set the timer for 20 minutes, turning pork halfway through cooking. Pork loin will be browned and have an internal temperature of at least 145°F when done. Serve warm.

PER SERVING

CALORIES: 249	FAT: 16g
PROTEIN: 24g	SODIUM: 278mg
FIBER: 0g	CARBOHYDRATES: 1g
NET CARBOHYDRATES: 1g	SUGAR: 0g

Bacon and Blue Cheese Burgers

Step up your weeknight dinner with this easy recipe that puts a tangy spin on traditional beef burgers. All the ingredients are mixed right in with the meat for delicious bacon and blue cheese flavor in each bite.

- **Pantry Staples: Salt, ground black pepper**
- **Hands-On Time: 10 minutes**
- **Cook Time: 15 minutes**

Serves 4

1 pound 70/30 ground beef

6 slices cooked sugar-free bacon, finely chopped

½ cup crumbled blue cheese

¼ cup peeled and chopped yellow onion

½ teaspoon salt

¼ teaspoon ground black pepper

1   In a large bowl, mix ground beef, bacon, blue cheese, and onion. Separate into four sections and shape each section into a patty. Sprinkle with salt and pepper.

2   Place patties into ungreased air fryer basket. Adjust the temperature to 350°F and set the timer for 15 minutes, turning patties halfway through cooking. Burgers will be done when internal temperature is at least 150°F for medium and 180°F for well. Serve warm.

PER SERVING

CALORIES: 319	FAT: 20g
PROTEIN: 28g	SODIUM: 785mg
FIBER: 0g	CARBOHYDRATES: 1g
NET CARBOHYDRATES: 1g	SUGAR: 1g

Blackened Steak Nuggets

Snack time couldn't be easier with these tender, flavorful bites. They cook up in less than 20 minutes and give you a low-carb protein boost to get through your day. For a special occasion, double or triple the recipe and serve with a chipotle mayonnaise dipping sauce.

- **Pantry Staples: Salt, ground black pepper, paprika, garlic powder**
- **Hands-On Time: 10 minutes**
- **Cook Time: 7 minutes**

Serves 2

1 pound rib eye steak, cut into 1" cubes

2 tablespoons salted butter, melted

½ teaspoon paprika

½ teaspoon salt

¼ teaspoon garlic powder

¼ teaspoon onion powder

¼ teaspoon ground black pepper

⅛ teaspoon cayenne pepper

1 Place steak into a large bowl and pour in butter. Toss to coat. Sprinkle with remaining ingredients.

2 Place bites into ungreased air fryer basket. Adjust the temperature to 400°F and set the timer for 7 minutes, shaking the basket three times during cooking. Steak will be crispy on the outside and browned when done and internal temperature is at least 150°F for medium and 180°F for well-done. Serve warm.

PER SERVING

CALORIES: 466	FAT: 28g
PROTEIN: 49g	SODIUM: 775mg
FIBER: 0g	CARBOHYDRATES: 1g
NET CARBOHYDRATES: 1g	SUGAR: 0g

Spinach and Provolone Steak Rolls

These steak rolls look impressive yet take just 10 minutes to prepare. The steak edges get dark brown while the inside can be cooked to your preferred doneness, similar to a quick sear on the stove.

- **Pantry Staples: Salt, ground black pepper**
- **Hands-On Time: 10 minutes**
- **Cook Time: 12 minutes**

Yields 8 rolls

- **1 (1-pound) flank steak, butterflied**
- **8 (1-ounce, ¼"-thick) deli slices provolone cheese**
- **1 cup fresh spinach leaves**
- **½ teaspoon salt**
- **¼ teaspoon ground black pepper**

CUSTOMIZE THEM!

Feel free to add your favorite fillings and seasonings to make these rolls your own. Switching out the cheese or even adding chopped sautéed vegetables will boost the flavor. Try chopped bell peppers and onions for fajita-flavored steak rolls.

1 Place steak on a large plate. Place provolone slices to cover steak, leaving 1" at the edges. Lay spinach leaves over cheese. Gently roll steak and tie with kitchen twine or secure with toothpicks. Carefully slice into eight pieces. Sprinkle each with salt and pepper.

2 Place rolls into ungreased air fryer basket, cut side up. Adjust the temperature to 400°F and set the timer for 12 minutes. Steak rolls will be browned and cheese will be melted when done and have an internal temperature of at least 150°F for medium steak and 180°F for well-done steak. Serve warm.

PER SERVING (2 ROLLS)

CALORIES: 376	**FAT:** 21g
PROTEIN: 40g	**SODIUM:** 844mg
FIBER: 0g	**CARBOHYDRATES:** 2g
NET CARBOHYDRATES: 2g	**SUGAR:** 0g

7

Fish and Seafood Main Dishes

Fish and seafood have huge appeal on the keto diet because they're one of the few proteins that are carb-free but still full of nutrients like omega-3 fatty acids. However, they can sometimes be difficult to cook because of how delicate they are. The good news is that your air fryer is able to handle the task perfectly and offer you evenly cooked seafood dishes in minutes.

Get ready to dive into the delicious seafood flavors of this chapter with everything from Bacon-Wrapped Scallops and Salmon Patties to Crab-Stuffed Avocado Boats and Fish Sticks! With just a few ingredients and simple instructions, you'll have a mouthwatering dish on the table in no time.

Salmon Patties

This recipe is a really great way to step up standard packaged salmon. You can serve these patties with tartar sauce or a drizzle of sriracha for a bit of heat. They're also handy for meal prepping—just double the recipe and store covered in the refrigerator for up to 4 days.

- Pantry Staples: None
- Hands-On Time: 5 minutes
- Cook Time: 8 minutes

Serves 4

12 ounces pouched pink salmon

3 tablespoons mayonnaise

⅓ cup blanched finely ground almond flour

½ teaspoon Cajun seasoning

1 medium avocado, peeled, pitted, and sliced

MAKE THESE PATTIES A FULL MEAL!

You can serve these patties on a bed of spinach, with a side of cauliflower rice, or between Cauliflower Buns (see recipe in Chapter 3) to enjoy it like a sandwich!

1 In a medium bowl, mix salmon, mayonnaise, flour, and Cajun seasoning. Form mixture into four patties.

2 Place patties into ungreased air fryer basket. Adjust the temperature to 400°F and set the timer for 8 minutes, turning patties halfway through cooking. Patties will be done when firm and golden brown.

3 Transfer patties to four medium plates and serve warm with avocado slices.

PER SERVING

CALORIES: 263	FAT: 18g
PROTEIN: 20g	SODIUM: 270mg
FIBER: 3g	CARBOHYDRATES: 5g
NET CARBOHYDRATES: 2g	SUGAR: 0g

Fish Sticks

Traditional fish sticks use carb-filled breading that doesn't usually have much flavor. This recipe adds flavor both in the low-carb coating and on the fish itself. Don't worry; you can still have tartar sauce—just be sure to watch for added sugar on the label.

- **Pantry Staples: None**
- **Hands-On Time: 15 minutes**
- **Cook Time: 12 minutes**

Serves 4

1 large egg
½ teaspoon Old Bay Seasoning
1½ ounces plain pork rinds, finely crushed
4 (4-ounce) cod fillets, cut into 1″ × 2″ sticks

THEY'RE KID FRIENDLY!

Ditch the high-carb traditional breaded fish sticks from the freezer aisle, and serve this delicious keto-friendly alternative that your kids won't be able to get enough of! You'll feel great knowing all the ingredients that were used, and you can even substitute a different fish, like haddock, if you prefer.

1 In a medium bowl, whisk egg. In a separate medium bowl, combine Old Bay Seasoning and pork rinds.

2 Dip each fish stick into egg, then gently press into pork rind mixture to coat all sides. Place fish sticks into ungreased air fryer basket. Adjust the temperature to 400°F and set the timer for 12 minutes, turning fish sticks halfway through cooking. Fish sticks will be golden brown and have an internal temperature of at least 145°F when done. Serve warm.

PER SERVING

CALORIES: 156	**FAT:** 5g
PROTEIN: 25g	**SODIUM:** 605mg
FIBER: 0g	**CARBOHYDRATES:** 0g
NET CARBOHYDRATES: 0g	**SUGAR:** 0g

Ahi Tuna Steaks

If you've never tried tuna steak, you're missing out! The fresh flavor is quite different from canned tuna, which is often made from a different species of tuna. Tuna steaks have a deep pink color and a lightly sweetened flavor.

- **Pantry Staples:** None
- **Hands-On Time:** 5 minutes
- **Cook Time:** 14 minutes

Serves 2

2 (6-ounce) ahi tuna steaks
2 tablespoons olive oil
3 tablespoons everything bagel seasoning

EVERYTHING BAGEL SEASONING

This seasoning blend is available in many grocery stores. It's commonly a mixture of salt, onion flakes, sesame seeds, and poppy seeds, which make it perfect for crusting tuna steaks (and saves you time spent mixing your own seasoning). Just be aware that it often already contains salt, so you won't need to add more.

1 Drizzle both sides of each steak with olive oil. Place seasoning on a medium plate and press each side of tuna steaks into seasoning to form a thick layer.

2 Place steaks into ungreased air fryer basket. Adjust the temperature to 400°F and set the timer for 14 minutes, turning steaks halfway through cooking. Steaks will be done when internal temperature is at least 145°F for well-done. Serve warm.

PER SERVING

CALORIES: 385	**FAT:** 14g
PROTEIN: 40g	**SODIUM:** 1,513mg
FIBER: 0g	**CARBOHYDRATES:** 0g
NET CARBOHYDRATES: 0g	**SUGAR:** 0g

5-Minute Shrimp

Shrimp is a simple seafood to cook, but it's even faster in the air fryer. Once it's prepared, you can do anything from serving it with a low-carb cocktail sauce to tossing it in a salad for a protein boost. Try sprinkling it with lemon pepper seasoning or your favorite herb blend before cooking.

- **Pantry Staples: Salt, ground black pepper**
- **Hands-On Time: 2 minutes**
- **Cook Time: 5 minutes**

Serves 4

1 pound medium shrimp, peeled and deveined

2 tablespoons salted butter, melted

¼ teaspoon salt

¼ teaspoon ground black pepper

1 In a large bowl, toss shrimp in butter, then sprinkle with salt and pepper.

2 Place shrimp into ungreased air fryer basket. Adjust the temperature to 400°F and set the timer for 5 minutes, shaking the basket halfway through cooking. Shrimp will be opaque and pink when done. Serve warm.

PER SERVING

CALORIES: 119

PROTEIN: 13g

FIBER: 0g

NET CARBOHYDRATES: 1g

FAT: 6g

SODIUM: 736mg

CARBOHYDRATES: 1g

SUGAR: 0g

Chili Lime Shrimp

When shrimp are cooked correctly, they form a perfect "C" shape and literally burst with flavor when you bite into them. When overcooked, they tend to curl into a tighter "C" shape or close into an "O" shape. It's easy to keep an eye on your shrimp in the air fryer to avoid overcooking and keep them juicy and delicious.

- Pantry Staples: Salt, ground black pepper, garlic powder
- Hands-On Time: 5 minutes
- Cook Time: 5 minutes

Serves 4

1 pound medium shrimp, peeled and deveined

1 tablespoon salted butter, melted

2 teaspoons chili powder

¼ teaspoon garlic powder

¼ teaspoon salt

¼ teaspoon ground black pepper

½ small lime, zested and juiced, divided

1 In a medium bowl, toss shrimp with butter, then sprinkle with chili powder, garlic powder, salt, pepper, and lime zest.

2 Place shrimp into ungreased air fryer basket. Adjust the temperature to 400°F and set the timer for 5 minutes. Shrimp will be firm and form a "C" shape when done.

3 Transfer shrimp to a large serving dish and drizzle with lime juice. Serve warm.

PER SERVING

CALORIES: 98		FAT: 4g	
PROTEIN: 13g		SODIUM: 752mg	
FIBER: 1g		CARBOHYDRATES: 2g	
NET CARBOHYDRATES: 1g		SUGAR: 0g	

MAKE A FILLING SHRIMP SALAD!

Make a salad with spinach and spring mix greens and top with these flavorful shrimp for a full, refreshing meal. Try adding tomatoes, onion, or cilantro as well. You can also top your salad with a creamy avocado dressing for added fat to round out the meal's macros.

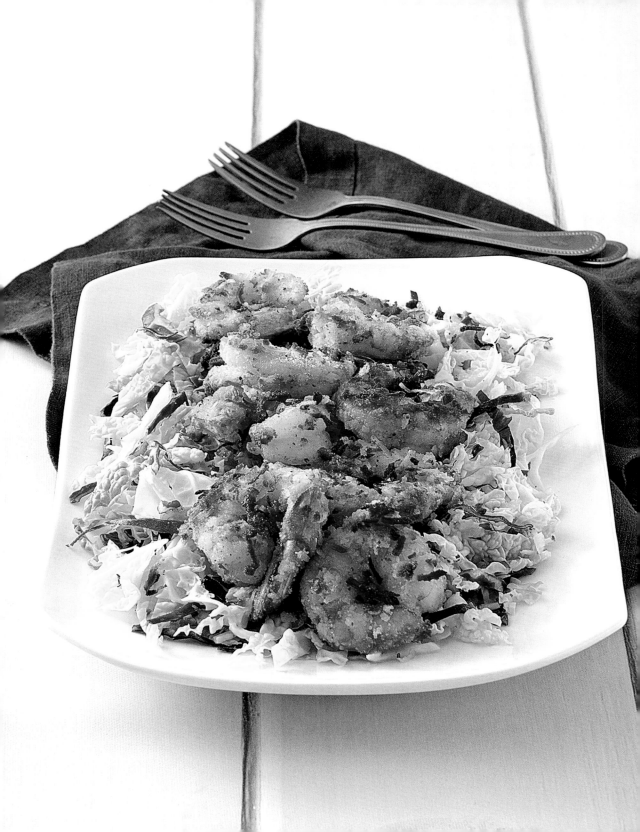

Crunchy Coconut Shrimp

Coconut flour is lower in carbs than other keto-friendly flours and thicker makes it the perfect breading for this recipe. The shredded coconut gets ilar to panko bread crumbs. Serve on a bed of spring salad mix to round _

- **Pantry Staples: None**
- **Hands-On Time: 5 minutes**
- **Cook Time: 8 minutes**

Serves 2

8 ounces jumbo shrimp, peeled and deveined

2 tablespoons salted butter, melted

½ teaspoon Old Bay Seasoning

¼ cup unsweetened shredded coconut

¼ cup coconut flour

1 In a large bowl, toss shrimp in butter and Old Bay Seasoning.

2 In a medium bowl, combine shredded coconut with coconut flour. Coat each piece of shrimp in coconut mixture.

3 Place shrimp into ungreased air fryer basket. Adjust the temperature to 400°F and set the timer for 8 minutes, gently turning shrimp halfway through cooking. Shrimp will be pink and C-shaped when done. Serve warm.

PER SERVING

CALORIES: 296	FAT: 19g
PROTEIN: 17g	SODIUM: 786mg
FIBER: 7g	CARBOHYDRATES: 13g
NET CARBOHYDRATES: 6g	SUGAR: 4g

Bacon-Wrapped Scallops

Scallops are a delicate mollusk that can be found at the fish stand in any grocery store. While they're traditionally panfried, preparing them in a controlled environment like the air fryer ensures a perfect cook. Serve with the Crispy Green Beans from Chapter 4 for a complete meal.

- **Pantry Staples: Salt, ground black pepper**
- **Hands-On Time: 5 minutes**
- **Cook Time: 10 minutes**

Serves 4

8 (1-ounce) sea scallops, cleaned and patted dry
8 slices sugar-free bacon
¼ teaspoon salt
¼ teaspoon ground black pepper

1 Wrap each scallop in 1 slice bacon and secure with a toothpick. Sprinkle with salt and pepper.

2 Place scallops into ungreased air fryer basket. Adjust the temperature to 360°F and set the timer for 10 minutes. Scallops will be opaque and firm, and have an internal temperature of 130°F when done. Serve warm.

PER SERVING

CALORIES: 125	FAT: 6g
PROTEIN: 14g	SODIUM: 691mg
FIBER: 0g	CARBOHYDRATES: 2g
NET CARBOHYDRATES: 2g	SUGAR: 0g

Garlic Lemon Scallops

Whipping up scallops at home can save money and give you better control over flavors. Lemon pairs well with garlic and adds a brightness to this buttery, tender dish. These scallops make a great appetizer or an extra-special seafood platter alongside crab legs and shrimp.

- **Pantry Staples: Salt, ground black pepper**
- **Hands-On Time: 5 minutes**
- **Cook Time: 10 minutes**

Serves 4

4 tablespoons salted butter, melted

4 teaspoons peeled and finely minced garlic

½ small lemon, zested and juiced

8 (1-ounce) sea scallops, cleaned and patted dry

¼ teaspoon salt

¼ teaspoon ground black pepper

1 In a small bowl, mix butter, garlic, lemon zest, and lemon juice. Place scallops in an ungreased 6" round nonstick baking dish. Pour butter mixture over scallops, then sprinkle with salt and pepper.

2 Place dish into air fryer basket. Adjust the temperature to 360°F and set the timer for 10 minutes. Scallops will be opaque and firm, and have an internal temperature of 130°F when done. Serve warm.

PER SERVING

CALORIES: 145	FAT: 11g
PROTEIN: 7g	SODIUM: 458mg
FIBER: 0g	CARBOHYDRATES: 3g
NET CARBOHYDRATES: 3g	SUGAR: 0g

Crab-Stuffed Avocado Boats

In just over 10 minutes, you can have an incredibly filling meal that's loaded with flavor. The warm avocado tastes and feels like a creamy sauce that goes perfectly with the sweet pieces of crab. You can use canned crab for this recipe to make it extra quick without sacrificing any flavor.

- **Pantry staples: None**
- **Hands-On Time: 5 minutes**
- **Cook Time: 7 minutes**

Serves 4

2 medium avocados, halved and pitted

8 ounces cooked crabmeat

¼ teaspoon Old Bay Seasoning

2 tablespoons peeled and diced yellow onion

2 tablespoons mayonnaise

1 Scoop out avocado flesh in each avocado half, leaving ½″ around edges to form a shell. Chop scooped-out avocado.

2 In a medium bowl, combine crabmeat, Old Bay Seasoning, onion, mayonnaise, and chopped avocado. Place ¼ mixture into each avocado shell.

3 Place avocado boats into ungreased air fryer basket. Adjust the temperature to 350°F and set the timer for 7 minutes. Avocado will be browned on the top and mixture will be bubbling when done. Serve warm.

PER SERVING

CALORIES: 209

PROTEIN: 12g

FIBER: 5g

NET CARBOHYDRATES: 1g

FAT: 15g

SODIUM: 307mg

CARBOHYDRATES: 6g

SUGAR: 0g

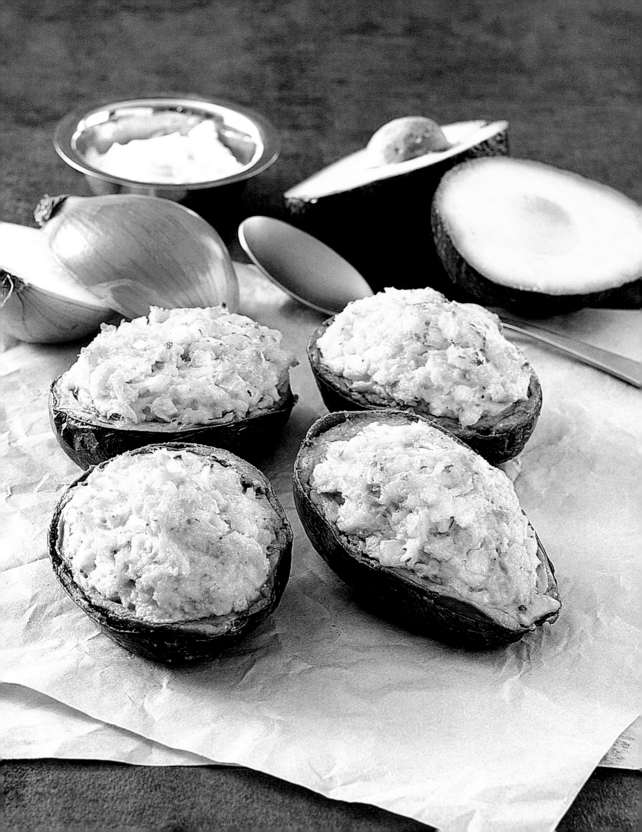

Lobster Tails

If you've been intimidated by the thought of cooking lobster tails, let the air fryer help you conquer your fear. You can enjoy these buttery, juicy lobster tails at home in less than 15 minutes, and with a few simple ingredients! Pair with Marinated Rib Eye (see recipe in Chapter 6) for a surf and turf night, or with Roasted Asparagus (see recipe in Chapter 4) for a balanced meal.

- **Pantry Staples: Salt, ground black pepper**
- **Hands-On Time: 5 minutes**
- **Cook Time: 9 minutes**

Serves 4

4 (6-ounce) lobster tails

2 tablespoons salted butter, melted

1 tablespoon peeled and finely minced garlic

¼ teaspoon salt

¼ teaspoon ground black pepper

2 tablespoons lemon juice

1 Carefully cut open lobster tails with scissors and pull back shell a little to expose meat. Pour butter over each tail, then sprinkle with garlic, salt, and pepper.

2 Place tails into ungreased air fryer basket. Adjust the temperature to 400°F and set the timer for 9 minutes. Lobster will be firm and opaque when done.

3 Transfer tails to four medium plates and pour lemon juice over lobster meat. Serve warm.

PER SERVING

CALORIES: 186	FAT: 7g
PROTEIN: 28g	SODIUM: 910mg
FIBER: 0g	CARBOHYDRATES: 1g
NET CARBOHYDRATES: 1g	SUGAR: 0g

PRESENTATION IS EVERYTHING

You can remove the tail meat completely or cook it inside of the shell, but one presentation method to help you flex your chef muscles is to "piggyback" the lobster tail. Cut a line down the shell, stopping at the fin, then remove the meat and set it on top of the shell to cook. It also helps prevent the tail from drying out when using quick cooking methods.

Tuna Cakes

This recipe is packed with protein and flavor. The air fryer also creates a delicious golden crust that adds texture. There are different flavored tuna pouches available that you can swap to make this dish your own—just be sure they don't have added sugars.

- **Pantry Staples: None**
- **Hands-On Time: 10 minutes**
- **Cook Time: 10 minutes**

Serves 4

4 (3-ounce) pouches tuna, drained

1 large egg, whisked

2 tablespoons peeled and chopped white onion

½ teaspoon Old Bay Seasoning

1 In a large bowl, mix all ingredients together and form into four patties.

2 Place patties into ungreased air fryer basket. Adjust the temperature to 400°F and set the timer for 10 minutes. Patties will be browned and crispy when done. Let cool 5 minutes before serving.

PER SERVING

CALORIES: 100
PROTEIN: 21g
FIBER: 0g
NET CARBOHYDRATES: 1g

FAT: 2g
SODIUM: 432mg
CARBOHYDRATES: 1g
SUGAR: 0g

Italian Baked Cod

Cod is delicate and mild in flavor, which is the perfect contrast to savory tomato sauce. The flavor from the sauce bakes into the fish in this recipe, so every bite is filled with delicious herbs. Pair with zucchini noodles for a fresh-tasting light meal.

- **Pantry Staples: Salt**
- **Hands-On Time: 5 minutes**
- **Cook Time: 12 minutes**

Serves 4

4 (6-ounce) cod fillets

2 tablespoons salted butter, melted

1 teaspoon Italian seasoning

¼ teaspoon salt

½ cup low-carb marinara sauce

1 Place cod into an ungreased 6″ round non-stick baking dish. Pour butter over cod and sprinkle with Italian seasoning and salt. Top with marinara.

2 Place dish into air fryer basket. Adjust the temperature to 350°F and set the timer for 12 minutes. Fillets will be lightly browned, easily flake, and have an internal temperature of at least 145°F when done. Serve warm.

PER SERVING

CALORIES: 193

PROTEIN: 27g

FIBER: 0g

NET CARBOHYDRATES: 2g

FAT: 8g

SODIUM: 811mg

CARBOHYDRATES: 2g

SUGAR: 1g

Mediterranean-Style Cod

This dish comes together quickly and with just a few ingredients, making it perfect for your weekly dinner plans. It's a light meal that uses Greek-inspired flavors to create a delicate, aromatic meal. The olives add a burst of salt that complements the natural sweetness of cod.

- **Pantry Staples: Salt**
- **Hands-On Time: 5 minutes**
- **Cook Time: 12 minutes**

Serves 4

4 (6-ounce) cod fillets

3 tablespoons fresh lemon juice

1 tablespoon olive oil

¼ teaspoon salt

6 cherry tomatoes, halved

¼ cup pitted and sliced kalamata olives

1 Place cod into an ungreased 6″ round non-stick baking dish. Pour lemon juice into dish and drizzle cod with olive oil. Sprinkle with salt. Place tomatoes and olives around baking dish in between fillets.

2 Place dish into air fryer basket. Adjust the temperature to 350°F and set the timer for 12 minutes, carefully turning cod halfway through cooking. Fillets will be lightly browned, easily flake, and have an internal temperature of at least 145°F when done. Serve warm.

PER SERVING

CALORIES: 189	FAT: 8g
PROTEIN: 26g	SODIUM: 891mg
FIBER: 0g	CARBOHYDRATES: 2g
NET CARBOHYDRATES: 2g	SUGAR: 1g

Rainbow Salmon Kebabs

These colorful kebabs are a playful take on regular fillets and have even more flavor. The vegetables get caramelized at the edges, cooking to a perfect tender crispness. This meal is also loaded with nutrients and heart-healthy fats that keep you going all day.

- **Pantry Staples: Salt, ground black pepper**
- **Hands-On Time: 10 minutes**
- **Cook Time: 8 minutes**

Serves 2

6 ounces boneless, skinless salmon, cut into 1" cubes

¼ medium red onion, peeled and cut into 1" pieces

½ medium yellow bell pepper, seeded and cut into 1" pieces

½ medium zucchini, trimmed and cut into ½" slices

1 tablespoon olive oil

½ teaspoon salt

¼ teaspoon ground black pepper

1 Using one 6" skewer, skewer 1 piece salmon, then 1 piece onion, 1 piece bell pepper, and finally 1 piece zucchini. Repeat this pattern with additional skewers to make four kebabs total. Drizzle with olive oil and sprinkle with salt and black pepper.

2 Place kebabs into ungreased air fryer basket. Adjust the temperature to 400°F and set the timer for 8 minutes, turning kebabs halfway through cooking. Salmon will easily flake and have an internal temperature of at least 145°F when done; vegetables will be tender. Serve warm.

PER SERVING

CALORIES: 183		**FAT:** 9g	
PROTEIN: 17g		**SODIUM:** 642mg	
FIBER: 1g		**CARBOHYDRATES:** 6g	
NET CARBOHYDRATES: 5g		**SUGAR:** 2g	

Spicy Fish Taco Bowl

This fresh-tasting dinner is perfect for when you want a light meal. The crispy cod makes a delicious bite paired with the creamy slaw. Feel free to add your own favorite taco bowl toppings such as diced avocado.

- **Pantry Staples: Salt, ground black pepper, garlic powder**
- **Hands-On Time: 10 minutes**
- **Cook Time: 12 minutes**

Serves 4

½ teaspoon salt
¼ teaspoon garlic powder
¼ teaspoon ground cumin
4 (4-ounce) cod fillets
4 cups finely shredded green cabbage
⅓ cup mayonnaise
¼ teaspoon ground black pepper
¼ cup chopped pickled jalapeños

1 Sprinkle salt, garlic powder, and cumin over cod and place into ungreased air fryer basket. Adjust the temperature to 350°F and set the timer for 12 minutes, turning fillets halfway through cooking. Cod will flake easily and have an internal temperature of at least 145°F when done.

2 In a large bowl, toss cabbage with mayonnaise, pepper, and jalapeños until fully coated. Serve cod warm over cabbage slaw on four medium plates.

PER SERVING

CALORIES: 221	**FAT:** 14g
PROTEIN: 18g	**SODIUM:** 850mg
FIBER: 2g	**CARBOHYDRATES:** 4g
NET CARBOHYDRATES: 2g	**SUGAR:** 2g

ADD A SPLASH OF LIME!
Adding a splash of fresh lime juice to the slaw and letting it chill for 10 minutes will brighten the flavors of the cabbage. The acidity from the lime mixed with the creamy mayonnaise takes this dish to the next level.

Cajun Salmon

Salmon is full of omega-3 fatty acids and other nutrients, but can be pricey to order in a restaurant. Making it at home will save money—and, in less than 15 minutes, dinner will be on the table. If you eat salmon only occasionally, you can even buy single servings and keep them frozen until ready to use.

- **Pantry Staples: Ground black pepper, paprika, garlic powder**
- **Hands-On Time: 5 minutes**
- **Cook Time: 7 minutes**

Serves 2

2 (4-ounce) boneless, skinless salmon fillets

2 tablespoons salted butter, softened

⅛ teaspoon cayenne pepper

½ teaspoon garlic powder

1 teaspoon paprika

¼ teaspoon ground black pepper

1 Brush both sides of each fillet with butter. In a small bowl, mix remaining ingredients and rub into fish on both sides.

2 Place fillets into ungreased air fryer basket. Adjust the temperature to 390°F and set the timer for 7 minutes. Internal temperature will be 145°F when done. Serve warm.

PER SERVING

CALORIES: 248
PROTEIN: 23g
FIBER: 1g
NET CARBOHYDRATES: 0g

FAT: 14g
SODIUM: 174mg
CARBOHYDRATES: 1g
SUGAR: 0g

Southern-Style Catfish

Buttermilk tends to have a higher ratio of carbs than is desired for a keto diet, but that doesn't mean you can't enjoy the creamy and tangy flavor. This recipe uses heavy whipping cream with a splash of lemon juice to mimic the taste of buttermilk with fewer carbs.

- **Pantry Staples: Salt, ground black pepper**
- **Hands-On Time: 10 minutes**
- **Cook Time: 12 minutes**

Serves 4

4 (7-ounce) catfish fillets

⅓ cup heavy whipping cream

1 tablespoon lemon juice

1 cup blanched finely ground almond flour

2 teaspoons Old Bay Seasoning

½ teaspoon salt

¼ teaspoon ground black pepper

1 Place catfish fillets into a large bowl with cream and pour in lemon juice. Stir to coat.

2 In a separate large bowl, mix flour and Old Bay Seasoning.

3 Remove each fillet and gently shake off excess cream. Sprinkle with salt and pepper. Press each fillet gently into flour mixture on both sides to coat.

4 Place fillets into ungreased air fryer basket. Adjust the temperature to 400°F and set the timer for 12 minutes, turning fillets halfway through cooking. Catfish will be golden brown and have an internal temperature of at least 145°F when done. Serve warm.

PER SERVING

CALORIES: 284

PROTEIN: 32g

FIBER: 1g

NET CARBOHYDRATES: 0g

FAT: 14g

SODIUM: 625mg

CARBOHYDRATES: 1g

SUGAR: 0g

Maple Butter Salmon

If you've been missing sticky-sweet glazes while on a keto diet, look no further than this recipe! It uses low-carb maple syrup and tangy mustard to create a sauce that's big on flavor but won't get you off track. For a bit of crunch, sprinkle sesame seeds over the fillets before cooking.

- **Pantry Staples: Salt**
- **Hands-On Time: 5 minutes**
- **Cook Time: 12 minutes**

Serves 4

2 tablespoons salted butter, melted

1 teaspoon low-carb maple syrup

1 teaspoon yellow mustard

4 (4-ounce) boneless, skinless salmon fillets

½ teaspoon salt

1 In a small bowl, whisk together butter, syrup, and mustard. Brush ½ mixture over each fillet on both sides. Sprinkle fillets with salt on both sides.

2 Place salmon into ungreased air fryer basket. Adjust the temperature to 400°F and set the timer for 12 minutes. Halfway through cooking, brush fillets on both sides with remaining syrup mixture. Salmon will easily flake and have an internal temperature of at least 145°F when done. Serve warm.

PER SERVING

CALORIES: 193

PROTEIN: 23g

FIBER: 0g

NET CARBOHYDRATES: 1g

SUGAR ALCOHOL: 0g

FAT: 9g

SODIUM: 435mg

CARBOHYDRATES: 1g

SUGAR: 0g

Crispy Parmesan Lobster Tails

These succulent lobster tails cook up just as quickly as you'll gobble them down! This recipe seasons the nutrient-rich lobster protein with just the right amount of spice to bring out the meat's natural flavors and impress any dinner guests!

- Pantry Staples: Salt, ground black pepper
- Hands-On Time: 5 minutes
- Cook Time: 7 minutes

Serves 4

4 (4-ounce) lobster tails

2 tablespoons salted butter, melted

1½ teaspoons Cajun seasoning, divided

¼ teaspoon salt

¼ teaspoon ground black pepper

¼ cup grated Parmesan cheese

½ ounce plain pork rinds, finely crushed

1   Cut lobster tails open carefully with a pair of scissors and gently pull meat away from shells, resting meat on top of shells.

2   Brush lobster meat with butter and sprinkle with 1 teaspoon Cajun seasoning, ¼ teaspoon per tail.

3   In a small bowl, mix remaining Cajun seasoning, salt, pepper, Parmesan, and pork rinds. Gently press ¼ mixture onto meat on each lobster tail.

4   Carefully place tails into ungreased air fryer basket. Adjust the temperature to 400°F and set the timer for 7 minutes. Lobster tails will be crispy and golden on top and have an internal temperature of at least 145°F when done. Serve warm.

PER SERVING

CALORIES: 184
PROTEIN: 23g
FIBER: 0g
NET CARBOHYDRATES: 1g

FAT: 9g
SODIUM: 931mg
CARBOHYDRATES: 1g
SUGAR: 0g

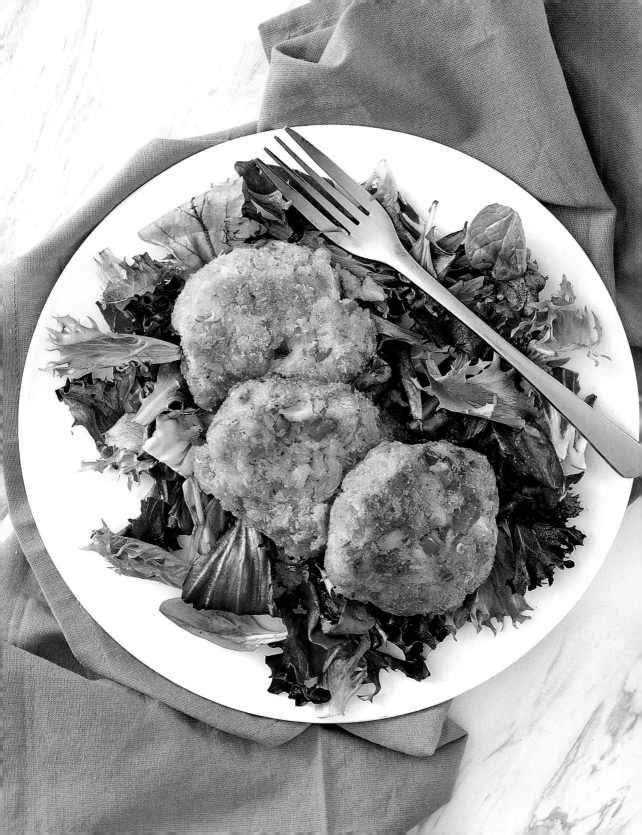

Crab Cakes

Traditionally, this recipe is made with flour or bread crumbs as a binder, but you'd be surprised how much better the natural flavor comes through without any fillers. Feel free to add your favorite crab cake mix-ins, such as chopped scallions, or a dash of cayenne pepper. These are great served on a bed of fresh salad leaves.

- **Pantry Staples: None**
- **Hands-On Time: 10 minutes**
- **Cook Time: 10 minutes**

Serves 4

8 ounces fresh lump
   crabmeat

2 tablespoons mayonnaise

1 teaspoon Old Bay
   Seasoning

½ ounce plain pork rinds,
   finely crushed

¼ cup seeded and chopped
   red bell pepper

1   In a large bowl, mix all ingredients together. Separate into four equal sections and form into patties.

2   Cut a piece of parchment to fit air fryer basket. Place patties onto ungreased parchment and into air fryer basket. Adjust the temperature to 380°F and set the timer for 10 minutes, turning patties halfway through cooking. Crab cakes will be golden when done. Serve warm.

PER SERVING

CALORIES: 116	FAT: 7g
PROTEIN: 12g	SODIUM: 561mg
FIBER: 0g	CARBOHYDRATES: 0g
NET CARBOHYDRATES: 0g	SUGAR: 0g

LUMP CRABMEAT

Lump crabmeat is made of larger pieces of crab and holds together better with fewer binders. If you want to save more money, you can also use canned meat—just be sure to drain it well first to avoid soggy cakes.

Snow Crab Legs

Snow crab legs are smaller and less expensive than king crab legs. They taste delicious dipped in butter, which makes them perfect for the keto diet, and with an air fryer you can have them ready in less than 30 minutes.

- **Pantry Staples: Coconut oil**
- **Hands-On Time: 5 minutes**
- **Cook Time: 15 minutes**

Serves 4

8 pounds fresh shell-on snow crab legs

2 tablespoons coconut oil

2 teaspoons Old Bay Seasoning

4 tablespoons salted butter, melted

2 teaspoons lemon juice

1 Place crab legs into ungreased air fryer basket, working in batches if needed. Drizzle legs with coconut oil and sprinkle with Old Bay Seasoning.

2 Adjust the temperature to 400°F and set the timer for 15 minutes, shaking the basket three times during cooking. Legs will turn a bright red-orange when done. Serve warm.

3 In a separate small bowl, whisk butter and lemon juice for dipping. Serve on the side.

PER SERVING

CALORIES: 284	**FAT:** 13g
PROTEIN: 38g	**SODIUM:** 1,186mg
FIBER: 0g	**CARBOHYDRATES:** 0g
NET CARBOHYDRATES: 0g	**SUGAR:** 0g

Lemon Butter Cod

This mild-tasting fish has a buttery texture that shines through with minimal ingredients. For this recipe, you'll use a baking dish; cod is delicate, and a dish will keep it from flaking apart and falling through the air fryer basket during removal.

- Pantry Staples: None
- Hands-On Time: 5 minutes
- Cook Time: 12 minutes

Serves 4

4 (4-ounce) cod fillets

2 tablespoons salted butter, melted

1 teaspoon Old Bay Seasoning

½ medium lemon, cut into 4 slices

1 Place cod fillets into an ungreased 6″ round nonstick baking dish. Brush tops of fillets with butter and sprinkle with Old Bay Seasoning. Lay 1 lemon slice on each fillet.

2 Cover dish with aluminum foil and place into air fryer basket. Adjust the temperature to 350°F and set the timer for 12 minutes, turning fillets halfway through cooking. Fish will be opaque and have an internal temperature of at least 145°F when done. Serve warm.

PER SERVING

CALORIES: 128

PROTEIN: 17g

FIBER: 0g

NET CARBOHYDRATES: 0g

FAT: 6g

SODIUM: 529mg

CARBOHYDRATES: 0g

SUGAR: 0g

Tuna-Stuffed Tomatoes

Tuna is a great inexpensive protein that you can keep on hand for snacks or quick meals. This recipe takes the idea of the classic tuna melt and gives it a low-carb twist. If you love flavored tuna pouches, feel free to use those in place of plain tuna for some extra flavor!

- **Pantry Staples: Salt, ground black pepper, coconut oil**
- **Hands-On Time: 5 minutes**
- **Cook Time: 5 minutes**

Serves 2

2 medium beefsteak tomatoes, tops removed, seeded, membranes removed

2 (2.6-ounce) pouches tuna packed in water, drained

1 medium stalk celery, trimmed and chopped

2 tablespoons mayonnaise

¼ teaspoon salt

¼ teaspoon ground black pepper

2 teaspoons coconut oil

¼ cup shredded mild Cheddar cheese

1 Scoop pulp out of each tomato, leaving ½" shell.

2 In a medium bowl, mix tuna, celery, mayonnaise, salt, and pepper. Drizzle with coconut oil. Spoon ½ mixture into each tomato and top each with 2 tablespoons Cheddar.

3 Place tomatoes into ungreased air fryer basket. Adjust the temperature to 320°F and set the timer for 5 minutes. Cheese will be melted when done. Serve warm.

PER SERVING

CALORIES: 219		**FAT:** 15g	
PROTEIN: 18g		**SODIUM:** 697mg	
FIBER: 1g		**CARBOHYDRATES:** 4g	
NET CARBOHYDRATES: 3g		**SUGAR:** 2g	

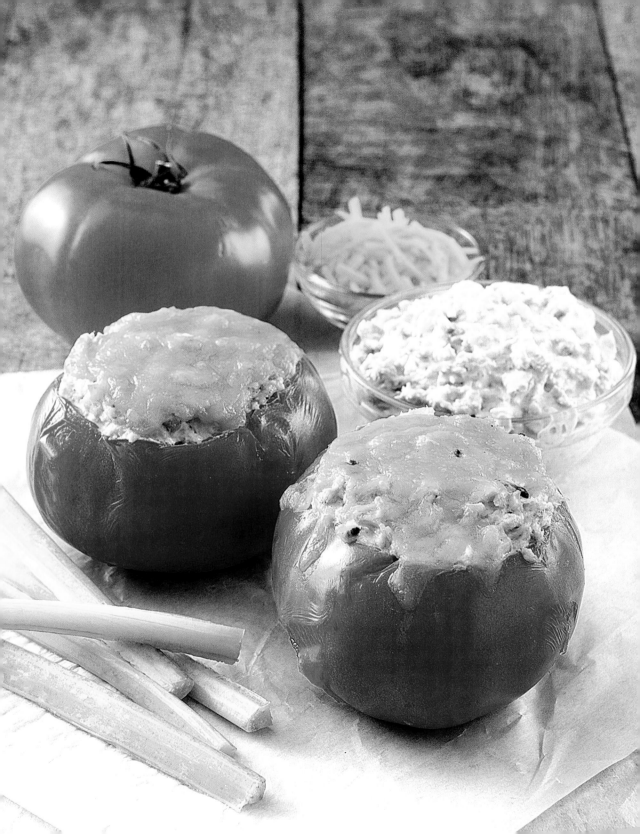

8

Vegetarian Main Dishes

Whether you are a vegetarian or are just looking to add more vegetables to your diet, you can use the air fryer to whip up easy meat-free meals with just a few ingredients and a few minutes of prep. It is especially important to include a lot of vegetables in your meals when eating a keto diet to ensure you are getting all of the necessary nutrients and balancing out the protein and fat. As a bonus, vegetarian dishes typically have fewer calories than meat options, so they are perfect for lighter meals.

Whatever your reasons for choosing vegetarian fare, this chapter has you covered! From Spinach and Artichoke–Stuffed Peppers and Mediterranean Pan Pizza to Pesto Vegetable Skewers and Stuffed Portobellos, these recipes will fill you up without depriving your taste buds!

Sweet Pepper Nachos

Mini sweet peppers are crunchy and delicious, with more nutritional value and fewer carbs than tortilla chips. Because of this, they're an excellent keto-friendly stand-in for when you're craving nachos.

- **Pantry Staples: None**
- **Hands-On Time: 10 minutes**
- **Cook Time: 5 minutes**

Serves 2

6 mini sweet peppers, seeded and sliced in half

¾ cup shredded Colby jack cheese

¼ cup sliced pickled jalapeños

½ medium avocado, peeled, pitted, and diced

2 tablespoons sour cream

WHERE TO FIND MINI SWEET PEPPERS

These peppers usually come in a bag in the refrigerated produce section of your local grocery store. You may also see a large bin with a variety of mini red, yellow, and orange peppers. If you have trouble finding them, look toward the salad bar—they're usually easy to spot.

1 Place peppers into an ungreased 6" round nonstick baking dish. Sprinkle with Colby and top with jalapeños.

2 Place dish into air fryer basket. Adjust the temperature to 350°F and set the timer for 5 minutes. Cheese will be melted and bubbly when done.

3 Remove dish from air fryer and top with avocado. Drizzle with sour cream. Serve warm.

PER SERVING

CALORIES: 310	**FAT:** 23g
PROTEIN: 12g	**SODIUM:** 440mg
FIBER: 5g	**CARBOHYDRATES:** 11g
NET CARBOHYDRATES: 6g	**SUGAR:** 4g

Spinach and Artichoke–Stuffed Peppers

Stuffed pepper recipes often call for rice, but filling them with a creamy spinach and artichoke dip is a low-carb way to serve a vegetarian dinner. This recipe calls for green bell peppers, but if you enjoy a sweeter crunch, you can swap for yellow or red bell peppers.

- **Pantry Staples: None**
- **Hands-On Time: 10 minutes**
- **Cook Time: 15 minutes**

Serves 4

2 ounces cream cheese, softened

½ cup shredded mozzarella cheese

½ cup chopped fresh spinach leaves

¼ cup chopped canned artichoke hearts

2 medium green bell peppers, halved and seeded

1 In a medium bowl, mix cream cheese, mozzarella, spinach, and artichokes. Spoon ¼ cheese mixture into each pepper half.

2 Place peppers into ungreased air fryer basket. Adjust the temperature to 320°F and set the timer for 15 minutes. Peppers will be tender and cheese will be bubbling and brown when done. Serve warm.

PER SERVING

CALORIES: 110
PROTEIN: 5g
FIBER: 2g
NET CARBOHYDRATES: 3g

FAT: 7g
SODIUM: 289mg
CARBOHYDRATES: 5g
SUGAR: 2g

Pesto Vegetable Skewers

These skewers are so fresh, satisfying, and loaded with nutrients that you won't miss the meat at all. They can be enjoyed as a main dish or in a half serving as a colorful side.

- **Pantry Staples: Salt, ground black pepper**
- **Hands-On Time: 40 minutes**
- **Cook Time: 8 minutes**

Yields 8 skewers

1 medium zucchini, trimmed and cut into ½" slices

½ medium yellow onion, peeled and cut into 1" squares

1 medium red bell pepper, seeded and cut into 1" squares

16 whole cremini mushrooms

⅓ cup basil pesto

½ teaspoon salt

¼ teaspoon ground black pepper

1 Divide zucchini slices, onion, and bell pepper into eight even portions. Place on 6" skewers for a total of eight kebabs. Add 2 mushrooms to each skewer and brush kebabs generously with pesto.

2 Sprinkle each kebab with salt and black pepper on all sides, then place into ungreased air fryer basket. Adjust the temperature to 375°F and set the timer for 8 minutes, turning kebabs halfway through cooking. Vegetables will be browned at the edges and tender-crisp when done. Serve warm.

PER SERVING (2 SKEWERS)

CALORIES: 107	FAT: 7g
PROTEIN: 4g	SODIUM: 500mg
FIBER: 2g	CARBOHYDRATES: 10g
NET CARBOHYDRATES: 8g	SUGAR: 4g

CUSTOM SKEWERS

Add your favorite vegetables to customize this meal! If there's one you don't like, swap it out for a favorite. Tomatoes, broccoli, and cauliflower all make great choices. You can also add a sprinkle of Italian seasoning for a pop of flavor!

Lemon Caper Cauliflower Steaks

Cauliflower is a mild vegetable that takes on any flavoring. This recipe uses capers for a tangy, salty punch that pairs wonderfully with the fresh lemon.

- **Pantry Staples: Salt, ground black pepper**
- **Hands-On Time: 5 minutes**
- **Cook Time: 15 minutes**

Serves 4

1 small head cauliflower, leaves and core removed, cut into 4 (½"-thick) "steaks"

4 tablespoons olive oil, divided

1 medium lemon, zested and juiced, divided

¼ teaspoon salt

⅛ teaspoon ground black pepper

1 tablespoon salted butter, melted

1 tablespoon capers, rinsed

1 Brush each cauliflower "steak" with ½ tablespoon olive oil on both sides and sprinkle with lemon zest, salt, and pepper on both sides.

2 Place cauliflower into ungreased air fryer basket. Adjust the temperature to 400°F and set the timer for 15 minutes, turning cauliflower halfway through cooking. Steaks will be golden at the edges and browned when done.

3 Transfer steaks to four medium plates. In a small bowl, whisk remaining olive oil, butter, lemon juice, and capers, and pour evenly over steaks. Serve warm.

PER SERVING

CALORIES: 162	FAT: 16g
PROTEIN: 1g	SODIUM: 238mg
FIBER: 1g	CARBOHYDRATES: 4g
NET CARBOHYDRATES: 3g	SUGAR: 1g

Crispy Eggplant Rounds

This breading, made from cheese crisps, makes this dish savory and delicious, whether it is your main entrée or a side. You can slice the eggplant with a knife, but a mandoline will give you perfectly even slices in a fraction of the time.

- **Pantry Staples: Salt, paprika, garlic powder**
- **Hands-On Time: 40 minutes**
- **Cook Time: 10 minutes**

Serves 4

1 large eggplant, ends trimmed, cut into ½" slices

½ teaspoon salt

2 ounces Parmesan 100% cheese crisps, finely ground

½ teaspoon paprika

¼ teaspoon garlic powder

1 large egg

1 Sprinkle eggplant rounds with salt. Place rounds on a kitchen towel for 30 minutes to draw out excess water. Pat rounds dry.

2 In a medium bowl, mix cheese crisps, paprika, and garlic powder. In a separate medium bowl, whisk egg. Dip each eggplant round in egg, then gently press into cheese crisps to coat both sides.

3 Place eggplant rounds into ungreased air fryer basket. Adjust the temperature to 400°F and set the timer for 10 minutes, turning rounds halfway through cooking. Eggplant will be golden and crispy when done. Serve warm.

PER SERVING

CALORIES: 93
PROTEIN: 7g
FIBER: 4g
NET CARBOHYDRATES: 5g

FAT: 4g
SODIUM: 484mg
CARBOHYDRATES: 9g
SUGAR: 5g

Cauliflower Rice–Stuffed Peppers

This light dinner is perfect for bringing to shared meals where you can show off how delicious the keto diet can be. The tomatoes soften to create a light sauce that gives the cauliflower rice extra flavor.

- **Pantry Staples: Salt, ground black pepper**
- **Hands-On Time: 10 minutes**
- **Cook Time: 15 minutes**

Serves 4

2 cups uncooked cauliflower rice

¾ cup drained canned petite diced tomatoes

2 tablespoons olive oil

1 cup shredded mozzarella cheese

¼ teaspoon salt

¼ teaspoon ground black pepper

4 medium green bell peppers, tops removed, seeded

1 In a large bowl, mix all ingredients except bell peppers. Scoop mixture evenly into peppers.

2 Place peppers into ungreased air fryer basket. Adjust the temperature to 350°F and set the timer for 15 minutes. Peppers will be tender and cheese will be melted when done. Serve warm.

PER SERVING

CALORIES: 185	**FAT:** 12g
PROTEIN: 9g	**SODIUM:** 403mg
FIBER: 4g	**CARBOHYDRATES:** 11g
NET CARBOHYDRATES: 7g	**SUGAR:** 6g

Mediterranean Pan Pizza

When you're in a hurry, or low on ingredients, this meal is as satisfying and delicious as a traditional pizza—without all the carbs. The vegetables on top are crisp, but if you like them extra soft, you can first sauté them on the stove until tender.

- **Pantry Staples: None**
- **Hands-On Time: 5 minutes**
- **Cook Time: 8 minutes**

Serves 2

1 cup shredded mozzarella cheese

¼ medium red bell pepper, seeded and chopped

½ cup chopped fresh spinach leaves

2 tablespoons chopped black olives

2 tablespoons crumbled feta cheese

1 Sprinkle mozzarella into an ungreased 6" round nonstick baking dish in an even layer. Add remaining ingredients on top.

2 Place dish into air fryer basket. Adjust the temperature to 350°F and set the timer for 8 minutes, checking halfway through to avoid burning. Top of pizza will be golden brown and the cheese melted when done.

3 Remove dish from fryer and let cool 5 minutes before slicing and serving.

PER SERVING

CALORIES: 215	FAT: 13g
PROTEIN: 16g	SODIUM: 541mg
FIBER: 0g	CARBOHYDRATES: 5g
NET CARBOHYDRATES: 5g	SUGAR: 2g

Vegetable Burgers

Many store-bought vegetable burgers use fillers or other ingredients that aren't keto friendly. These burgers are made with whole, low-carb ingredients. You can enjoy them as bunless patties or in lettuce as wraps with crisp red onion and creamy avocado slices. You can also make them sliders—just take 2 minutes off the cooking time.

- **Pantry Staples: Salt, ground black pepper**
- **Hands-On Time: 10 minutes**
- **Cook Time: 12 minutes**

Serves 4

8 ounces cremini mushrooms

2 large egg yolks

½ medium zucchini, trimmed and chopped

¼ cup peeled and chopped yellow onion

1 clove garlic, peeled and finely minced

½ teaspoon salt

¼ teaspoon ground black pepper

1 Place all ingredients into a food processor and pulse twenty times until finely chopped and combined.

2 Separate mixture into four equal sections and press each into a burger shape. Place burgers into ungreased air fryer basket. Adjust the temperature to 375°F and set the timer for 12 minutes, turning burgers halfway through cooking. Burgers will be browned and firm when done.

3 Place burgers on a large plate and let cool 5 minutes before serving.

PER SERVING

CALORIES: 48	**FAT:** 2g
PROTEIN: 3g	**SODIUM:** 299mg
FIBER: 1g	**CARBOHYDRATES:** 5g
NET CARBOHYDRATES: 4g	**SUGAR:** 2g

Stuffed Portobellos

These cheesy mushrooms are filled with colorful vegetables and loaded with nutrients. The edges of the mushrooms get crispy while leaving the insides tender but firm. They are surprisingly filling and also work great as a snack!

- **Pantry Staples: Salt, coconut oil**
- **Hands-On Time: 10 minutes**
- **Cook Time: 8 minutes**

Serves 4

3 ounces cream cheese, softened

½ medium zucchini, trimmed and chopped

¼ cup seeded and chopped red bell pepper

1½ cups chopped fresh spinach leaves

4 large portobello mushrooms, stems removed

2 tablespoons coconut oil, melted

½ teaspoon salt

1 In a medium bowl, mix cream cheese, zucchini, pepper, and spinach.

2 Drizzle mushrooms with coconut oil and sprinkle with salt. Scoop ¼ zucchini mixture into each mushroom.

3 Place mushrooms into ungreased air fryer basket. Adjust the temperature to 400°F and set the timer for 8 minutes. Portobellos will be tender and tops will be browned when done. Serve warm.

PER SERVING

CALORIES: 158		FAT: 13g	
PROTEIN: 4g		SODIUM: 386mg	
FIBER: 2g		CARBOHYDRATES: 6g	
NET CARBOHYDRATES: 4g		SUGAR: 4g	

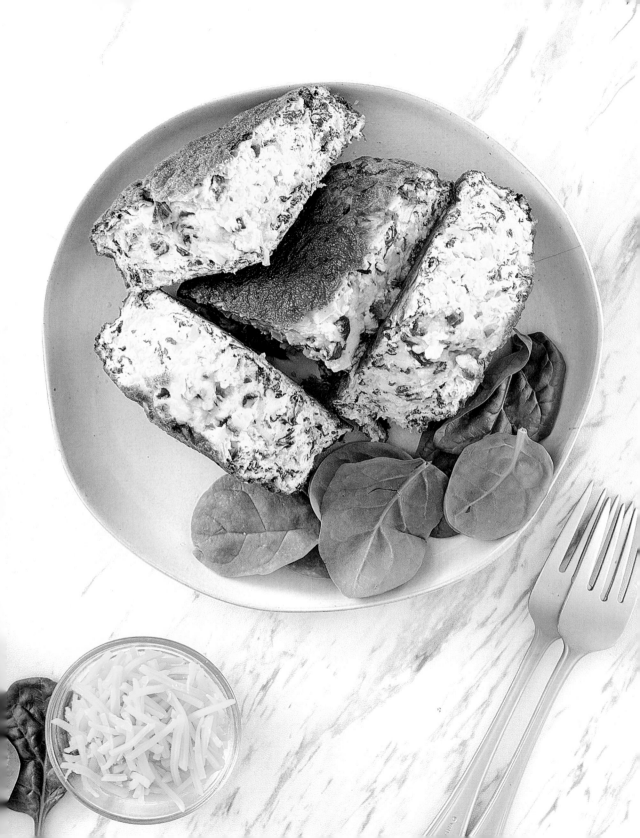

Crustless Spinach and Cheese Frittata

This meal is packed with protein to keep you full all day. Feel free to customize with your favorite vegetables, especially if you have leftovers to use up, like cooked asparagus or mushrooms. Just chop them up and toss them in the egg mixture before air frying.

- **Pantry Staples: Salt, ground black pepper**
- **Hands-On Time: 10 minutes**
- **Cook Time: 20 minutes**

Serves 4

6 large eggs

½ cup heavy whipping cream

1 cup frozen chopped spinach, drained

1 cup shredded sharp Cheddar cheese

¼ cup peeled and diced yellow onion

½ teaspoon salt

¼ teaspoon ground black pepper

1 In a large bowl, whisk eggs and cream together. Whisk in spinach, Cheddar, onion, salt, and pepper.

2 Pour mixture into an ungreased 6" round nonstick baking dish. Place dish into air fryer basket. Adjust the temperature to 320°F and set the timer for 20 minutes. Eggs will be firm and slightly browned when done. Serve immediately.

PER SERVING

CALORIES: 339	FAT: 25g
PROTEIN: 18g	SODIUM: 619mg
FIBER: 1g	CARBOHYDRATES: 4g
NET CARBOHYDRATES: 3g	SUGAR: 2g

ower Pizza Crust

sts that advertise as low-carb often still utilize fillers that aren't ideal for a
ng your crusts at home, you have total control of what goes into them.
complete your pizza, simply cook the crust, then add toppings and air fry at 350°F for
3 minutes.

- **Pantry Staples: None**
- **Hands-On Time: 20 minutes**
- **Cook Time: 7 minutes**

Serves 2

1 (12-ounce) steamer bag
   cauliflower, cooked
   according to package
   instructions
½ cup shredded sharp
   Cheddar cheese
1 large egg
2 tablespoons blanched
   finely ground almond
   flour
1 teaspoon Italian seasoning

CRUST COSTS

There are store-bought frozen cauliflower crusts that are keto friendly and work in a pinch; however, they can cost up to $10. You can usually find a steamer bag of cauliflower for around $1 to make your own.

1 Let cooked cauliflower cool for 10 minutes. Using a kitchen towel, wring out excess moisture from cauliflower and place into food processor.

2 Add Cheddar, egg, flour, and Italian seasoning to processor and pulse ten times until cauliflower is smooth and all ingredients are combined.

3 Cut two pieces of parchment paper to fit air fryer basket. Divide cauliflower mixture into two equal portions and press each into a 6" round on ungreased parchment.

4 Place crusts on parchment into air fryer basket. Adjust the temperature to 360°F and set the timer for 7 minutes, gently turning crusts halfway through cooking.

5 Store crusts in refrigerator in an airtight container up to 4 days or freeze between sheets of parchment in a sealable storage bag for up to 2 months.

PER SERVING

CALORIES: 233	**FAT:** 14g
PROTEIN: 15g	**SODIUM:** 257mg
FIBER: 5g	**CARBOHYDRATES:** 10g
NET CARBOHYDRATES: 5g	**SUGAR:** 4g

Roasted Spaghetti Squash

The results are worth the extra bit of cooking time, because roasting brings out the natural sweetness of the spaghetti squash, which is a great complement to the acidity of low-carb marinara.

- **Pantry Staples: Garlic powder, coconut oil**
- **Hands-On Time: 10 minutes**
- **Cook Time: 45 minutes**

Serves 6

1 (4-pound) spaghetti squash, halved and seeded

2 tablespoons coconut oil

4 tablespoons salted butter, melted

1 teaspoon garlic powder

2 teaspoons dried parsley

1 Brush shell of spaghetti squash with coconut oil. Brush inside with butter. Sprinkle inside with garlic powder and parsley.

2 Place squash skin side down into ungreased air fryer basket, working in batches if needed. Adjust the temperature to 350°F and set the timer for 30 minutes. When the timer beeps, flip squash and cook an additional 15 minutes until fork-tender.

3 Use a fork to remove spaghetti strands from shell and serve warm.

PER SERVING

CALORIES: 104		**FAT:** 7g	
PROTEIN: 1g		**SODIUM:** 84mg	
FIBER: 2g		**CARBOHYDRATES:** 9g	
NET CARBOHYDRATES: 7g		**SUGAR:** 3g	

MEAL PREP SQUASH

Spaghetti squash is a versatile option for meal prep. You can add your favorite sauces and cooked proteins, or turn it into a stir-fry to keep meals from getting boring. Store cooked spaghetti squash in the refrigerator for up to 4 days.

Alfredo Eggplant Stacks

These creamy stacks are loaded with fat to keep you full and satisfied! The tomato adds the perfect amount of acidity to complement the naturally keto-friendly Alfredo sauce.

- **Pantry Staples: None**
- **Hands-On Time: 5 minutes**
- **Cook Time: 12 minutes**

Serves 6

1 large eggplant, ends trimmed, cut into ¼" slices

1 medium beefsteak tomato, cored and cut into ¼" slices

1 cup Alfredo sauce

8 ounces fresh mozzarella cheese, cut into 18 slices

2 tablespoons fresh parsley leaves

1 Place 6 slices eggplant in bottom of an ungreased 6" round nonstick baking dish. Place 1 slice tomato on top of each eggplant round, followed by 1 tablespoon Alfredo and 1 slice mozzarella. Repeat with remaining ingredients, about three repetitions.

2 Cover dish with aluminum foil and place dish into air fryer basket. Adjust the temperature to 350°F and set the timer for 12 minutes. Eggplant will be tender when done.

3 Sprinkle parsley evenly over each stack. Serve warm.

PER SERVING

CALORIES: 173	**FAT:** 10g
PROTEIN: 10g	**SODIUM:** 506mg
FIBER: 3g	**CARBOHYDRATES:** 9g
NET CARBOHYDRATES: 6g	**SUGAR:** 5g

White Cheddar and Mushroom Soufflés

This recipe uses whipped egg whites to make a fluffy and delicious meal for any occasion. You can beat them by hand, but an electric mixer makes things a little faster. You can also use chopped chives as a garnish for a fresh taste that isn't overpowering.

- **Pantry Staples: Salt, ground black pepper**
- **Hands-On Time: 15 minutes**
- **Cook Time: 12 minutes**

Serves 4

3 large eggs, whites and yolks separated

½ cup sharp white Cheddar cheese

3 ounces cream cheese, softened

¼ teaspoon cream of tartar

¼ teaspoon salt

¼ teaspoon ground black pepper

½ cup cremini mushrooms, sliced

1 In a large bowl, whip egg whites until stiff peaks form, about 2 minutes. In a separate large bowl, beat Cheddar, egg yolks, cream cheese, cream of tartar, salt, and pepper together until combined.

2 Fold egg whites into cheese mixture, being careful not to stir. Fold in mushrooms, then pour mixture evenly into four ungreased 4" ramekins.

3 Place ramekins into air fryer basket. Adjust the temperature to 350°F and set the timer for 12 minutes. Eggs will be browned on the top and firm in the center when done. Serve warm.

PER SERVING

CALORIES: 185	FAT: 14g
PROTEIN: 10g	SODIUM: 367mg
FIBER: 0g	CARBOHYDRATES: 2g
NET CARBOHYDRATES: 2g	SUGAR: 1g

Cheesy Broccoli Sticks

Broccoli is full of vitamins, and though it doesn't get the same attention as cauliflower, it's just as versatile. This meal has all the flavors of broccoli Cheddar soup in a crispy, handheld version.

- **Pantry Staples: Salt**
- **Hands-On Time: 10 minutes**
- **Cook Time: 16 minutes**

Serves 2

1 (10-ounce) steamer bag broccoli florets, cooked according to package instructions

1 large egg

1 ounce Parmesan 100% cheese crisps, finely ground

½ cup shredded sharp Cheddar cheese

½ teaspoon salt

½ cup ranch dressing

1 Let cooked broccoli cool 5 minutes, then place into a food processor with egg, cheese crisps, Cheddar, and salt. Process on low for 30 seconds until all ingredients are combined and begin to stick together.

2 Cut a sheet of parchment paper to fit air fryer basket. Take one scoop of mixture, about 3 tablespoons, and roll into a 4" stick shape, pressing down gently to flatten the top. Place stick on ungreased parchment into air fryer basket. Repeat with remaining mixture to form eight sticks.

3 Adjust the temperature to 350°F and set the timer for 16 minutes, turning sticks halfway through cooking. Sticks will be golden brown when done.

4 Serve warm with ranch dressing on the side for dipping.

PER SERVING

CALORIES: 242
PROTEIN: 18g
FIBER: 4g
NET CARBOHYDRATES: 4g

FAT: 15g
SODIUM: 1,039mg
CARBOHYDRATES: 8g
SUGAR: 2g

Zucchini Fritters

This recipe keeps the zucchini flavor front and center with just a few simple ingredients to help enhance its flavor. Feel free to make it your own by adding shredded carrots or your favorite vegetable seasoning.

- **Pantry Staples: Salt, garlic powder**
- **Hands-On Time: 45 minutes**
- **Cook Time: 12 minutes**

Serves 4

1½ medium zucchini, trimmed and grated
½ teaspoon salt, divided
1 large egg, whisked
¼ teaspoon garlic powder
¼ cup grated Parmesan cheese

1 Place grated zucchini on a kitchen towel and sprinkle with ¼ teaspoon salt. Wrap in towel and let sit 30 minutes, then wring out as much excess moisture as possible.

2 Place zucchini into a large bowl and mix with egg, remaining salt, garlic powder, and Parmesan. Cut a piece of parchment to fit air fryer basket. Divide mixture into four mounds, about ⅓ cup each, and press out into 4″ rounds on ungreased parchment.

3 Place parchment with rounds into air fryer basket. Adjust the temperature to 400°F and set the timer for 12 minutes, turning fritters halfway through cooking. Fritters will be crispy on the edges and tender but firm in the center when done. Serve warm.

PER SERVING

CALORIES: 56	**FAT:** 3g
PROTEIN: 4g	**SODIUM:** 426mg
FIBER: 1g	**CARBOHYDRATES:** 3g
NET CARBOHYDRATES: 2g	**SUGAR:** 2g

Pesto Spinach Flatbread

This recipe makes a crust that's creamy on the inside and crispy on the outside. You won't even need extra cheese on top, because the delicious crust gives you just the perfect amount of flavor to complement the pesto.

- **Pantry Staples: None**
- **Hands-On Time: 10 minutes**
- **Cook Time: 8 minutes**

Serves 4

1 cup blanched finely ground almond flour

2 ounces cream cheese

2 cups shredded mozzarella cheese

1 cup chopped fresh spinach leaves

2 tablespoons basil pesto

BALANCE IT OUT WITH A SALAD!

This dish is full of fat, which makes it delicious but also a little dense. A salad with mixed greens, nuts, and strawberries would be an excellent side to balance out the meal and help you get in more fiber!

1 Place flour, cream cheese, and mozzarella in a large microwave-safe bowl and microwave on high 45 seconds, then stir.

2 Fold in spinach and microwave an additional 15 seconds. Stir until a soft dough ball forms.

3 Cut two pieces of parchment paper to fit air fryer basket. Separate dough into two sections and press each out on ungreased parchment to create 6" rounds.

4 Spread 1 tablespoon pesto over each flatbread and place rounds on parchment into ungreased air fryer basket. Adjust the temperature to 350°F and set the timer for 8 minutes, turning crusts halfway through cooking. Flatbread will be golden when done.

5 Let cool 5 minutes before slicing and serving.

PER SERVING

CALORIES: 414	FAT: 31g
PROTEIN: 21g	SODIUM: 517mg
FIBER: 3g	CARBOHYDRATES: 10g
NET CARBOHYDRATES: 7g	SUGAR: 3g

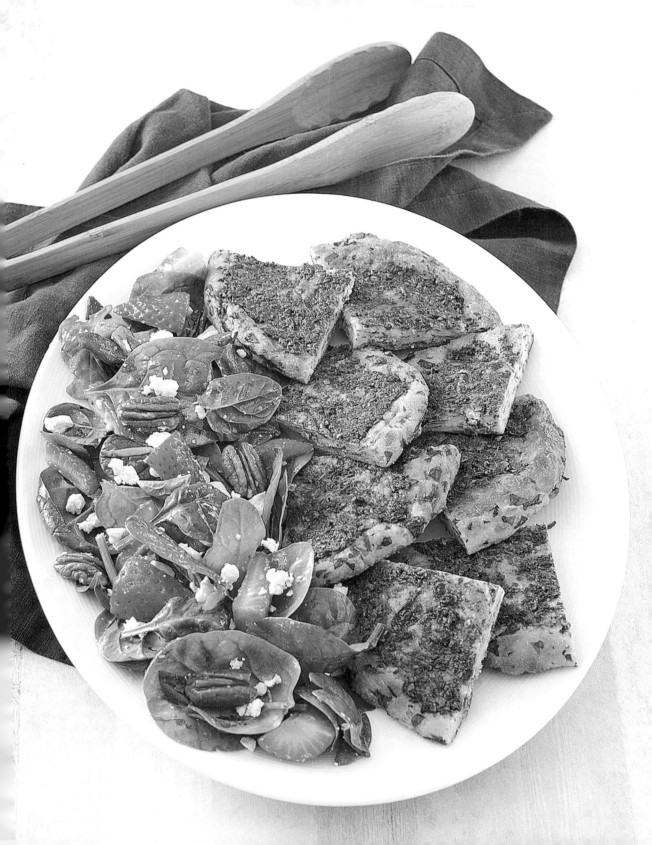

Savory Herb Cloud Eggs

This isn't your typical egg dish. The whipped egg whites form a golden brown and crispy bed for the herb-covered, creamy yolk. Though it's simple and made with just a few ingredients, the texture elevates the dish and turns it into something worthy of a Sunday brunch with friends.

- **Pantry Staples: Salt**
- **Hands-On Time: 5 minutes**
- **Cook Time: 8 minutes**

Serves 2

2 large eggs, whites and yolks separated

¼ teaspoon salt

¼ teaspoon dried oregano

2 tablespoons chopped fresh chives

2 teaspoons salted butter, melted

1 In a large bowl, whip egg whites until stiff peaks form, about 3 minutes. Place egg whites evenly into two ungreased 4" ramekins. Sprinkle evenly with salt, oregano, and chives. Place 1 whole egg yolk in center of each ramekin and drizzle with butter.

2 Place ramekins into air fryer basket. Adjust the temperature to 350°F and set the timer for 8 minutes. Egg whites will be fluffy and browned when done. Serve warm.

PER SERVING

CALORIES: 105

PROTEIN: 6g

FIBER: 0g

NET CARBOHYDRATES: 1g

FAT: 8g

SODIUM: 391mg

CARBOHYDRATES: 1g

SUGAR: 0g

Crispy Cabbage Steaks

This dish uses a few simple herbs to enhance the flavor of the roasted cabbage. The cabbage is crispy around the edges and tender in the center, which gives it a perfect balance. You can perk it up with a drizzle of your favorite vinegar-based dressing for added tang.

- Pantry Staples: Salt, ground black pepper
- Hands-On Time: 5 minutes
- Cook Time: 10 minutes

Serves 4

1 small head green cabbage, cored and cut into ½"-thick slices
¼ teaspoon salt
¼ teaspoon ground black pepper
2 tablespoons olive oil
1 clove garlic, peeled and finely minced
½ teaspoon dried thyme
½ teaspoon dried parsley

1 Sprinkle each side of cabbage with salt and pepper, then place into ungreased air fryer basket, working in batches if needed.

2 Drizzle each side of cabbage with olive oil, then sprinkle with remaining ingredients on both sides. Adjust the temperature to 350°F and set the timer for 10 minutes, turning "steaks" halfway through cooking. Cabbage will be browned at the edges and tender when done. Serve warm.

PER SERVING

CALORIES: 105
PROTEIN: 2g
FIBER: 5g
NET CARBOHYDRATES: 6g

FAT: 7g
SODIUM: 177mg
CARBOHYDRATES: 11g
SUGAR: 6g

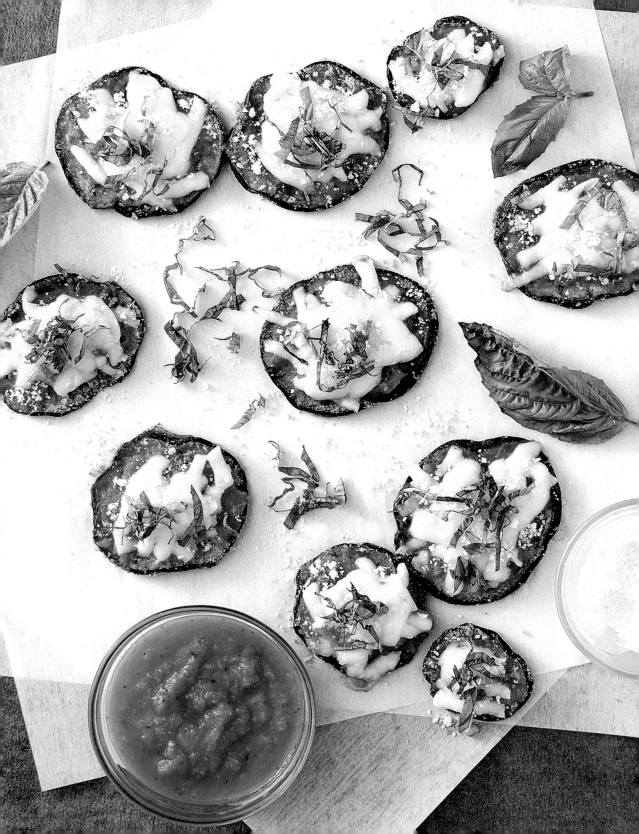

Eggplant Parmesan

This comfort food is quick and easy to make in the air fryer. The crispy eggplant slices are covered in sauce and gooey melted cheese for the ultimate filling entrée. Add strips of fresh basil leaves and freshly grated Parmesan as garnish to take this savory dish to the next level.

- **Pantry Staples:** Salt, coconut oil
- **Hands-On Time:** 40 minutes
- **Cook Time:** 17 minutes

Serves 4

1 medium eggplant, ends trimmed, sliced into ½" rounds

¼ teaspoon salt

2 tablespoons coconut oil

½ cup grated Parmesan cheese

1 ounce 100% cheese crisps, finely crushed

½ cup low-carb marinara sauce

½ cup shredded mozzarella cheese

LOW-CARB MARINARA

Invest some time in reading the nutrition labels before reaching for your favorite sauce! Tomato has natural sugars that can't be avoided, but many brands pile on added sugars. Try to stay around 4g net carbs per serving of marinara to better stay on track.

1 Sprinkle eggplant rounds with salt on both sides and wrap in a kitchen towel for 30 minutes. Press to remove excess water, then drizzle rounds with coconut oil on both sides.

2 In a medium bowl, mix Parmesan and cheese crisps. Press each eggplant slice into mixture to coat both sides.

3 Place rounds into ungreased air fryer basket. Adjust the temperature to 350°F and set the timer for 15 minutes, turning rounds halfway through cooking. They will be crispy around the edges when done.

4 When timer beeps, spoon marinara over rounds and sprinkle with mozzarella. Continue cooking an additional 2 minutes at 350°F until cheese is melted. Serve warm.

PER SERVING

CALORIES: 255	FAT: 17g
PROTEIN: 11g	SODIUM: 658mg
FIBER: 4g	CARBOHYDRATES: 12g
NET CARBOHYDRATES: 8g	SUGAR: 6g

9

Desserts

Who doesn't love dessert? Unfortunately, because traditional flours and sugars don't fit into a keto diet, it can sometimes feel impossible to find a mouthwatering treat that will satisfy your sweet tooth without compromising your health goals. Thankfully, there are a ton of keto options out there to keep you on track. And with the air fryer, you're able create a wide range of perfectly portioned, keto-friendly sweets that always hit the spot.

This chapter makes dessert time extra easy! With just a few ingredients and simple steps, these guilt-free goodies can be on your table (or in your stomach) in no time. From Peanut Butter Cookies and Easy Keto Danish to Chilled Strawberry Pie and Chocolate Lava Cakes, there's a recipe to satisfy every craving!

Mini Crustless Peanut Butter Cheesecake

This creamy and nutty dessert proves that you don't need a crust to make a perfect cheesecake! Though it's portioned for two small servings, you can certainly double (or triple) the recipe based on the size of your pans and air fryer.

- **Pantry Staples: Vanilla extract**
- **Hands-On Time: 10 minutes**
- **Cook Time: 10 minutes**

Serves 2

4 ounces cream cheese, softened

2 tablespoons confectioners' erythritol

1 tablespoon all-natural, no-sugar-added peanut butter

½ teaspoon vanilla extract

1 large egg, whisked

1 In a medium bowl, mix cream cheese and erythritol until smooth. Add peanut butter and vanilla, mixing until smooth. Add egg and stir just until combined.

2 Spoon mixture into an ungreased 4″ springform nonstick pan and place into air fryer basket. Adjust the temperature to 300°F and set the timer for 10 minutes. Edges will be firm, but center will be mostly set with only a small amount of jiggle when done.

3 Let pan cool at room temperature 30 minutes, cover with plastic wrap, then place into refrigerator at least 2 hours. Serve chilled.

PER SERVING

CALORIES: 282	**FAT:** 23g
PROTEIN: 9g	**SODIUM:** 242mg
FIBER: 1g	**CARBOHYDRATES:** 13g
NET CARBOHYDRATES: 3g	**SUGAR:** 2g
SUGAR ALCOHOL: 9g	

Pecan Snowball Cookies

These are some of the easiest cookies you'll ever make! Perfect for bringing to holiday gatherings, or just snacking on something sweet, they'll soon become a favorite. As they cool, the outside gets crispy while the inside stays soft, with a nice crunch from the pecans.

- **Pantry Staples: Vanilla extract**
- **Hands-On Time: 5 minutes**
- **Cook Time: 24 minutes**

Yields 12 cookies

1 cup chopped pecans
½ cup salted butter, melted
½ cup coconut flour
¾ cup confectioners' erythritol, divided
1 teaspoon vanilla extract

1 In a food processor, blend together pecans, butter, flour, ½ cup erythritol, and vanilla 1 minute until a dough forms.

2 Form dough into twelve individual cookie balls, about 1 tablespoon each.

3 Cut three pieces of parchment to fit air fryer basket. Place four cookies on each ungreased parchment and place one piece parchment with cookies into air fryer basket. Adjust air fryer temperature to 325°F and set the timer for 8 minutes. Repeat cooking with remaining batches.

4 When the timer goes off, allow cookies to cool 5 minutes on a large serving plate until cool enough to handle. While still warm, dust cookies with remaining erythritol. Allow to cool completely, about 15 minutes, before serving.

PER SERVING (1 COOKIE)

CALORIES: 151	**FAT:** 14g
PROTEIN: 2g	**SODIUM:** 64mg
FIBER: 3g	**CARBOHYDRATES:** 13g
NET CARBOHYDRATES: 1g	**SUGAR:** 1g
SUGAR ALCOHOL: 9g	

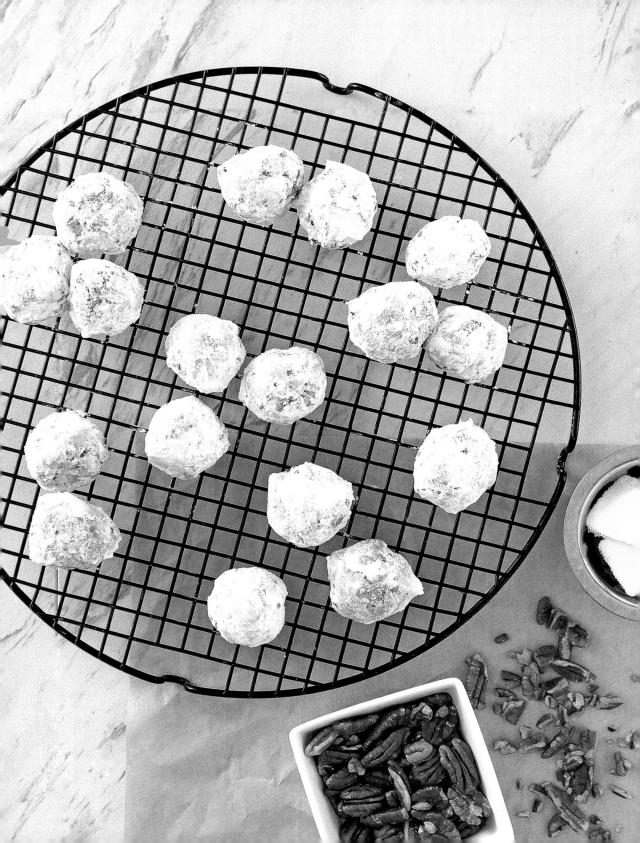

Chocolate Doughnut Holes

Flavored protein powders not only add protein to baked goods but also enhance the texture and give them a better rise. These doughnut holes will taste like the protein powder you use, so pick a low-carb flavor you enjoy. Quest Nutrition has a variety of keto-friendly flavors such as Vanilla Milkshake and Cinnamon Crunch.

- **Pantry Staples: Baking powder, vanilla extract**
- **Hands-On Time: 10 minutes**
- **Cook Time: 6 minutes**

Yields 20 doughnut holes

1 cup blanched finely ground almond flour
½ cup low-carb vanilla protein powder
½ cup granular erythritol
¼ cup unsweetened cocoa powder
½ teaspoon baking powder
2 large eggs, whisked
½ teaspoon vanilla extract

1 Mix all ingredients in a large bowl until a soft dough forms. Separate and roll dough into twenty balls, about 2 tablespoons each.

2 Cut a piece of parchment to fit your air fryer basket. Working in batches if needed, place doughnut holes into air fryer basket on ungreased parchment. Adjust the temperature to 380°F and set the timer for 6 minutes, flipping doughnut holes halfway through cooking. Doughnut holes will be golden and firm when done. Let cool completely before serving, about 10 minutes.

PER SERVING (2 DOUGHNUT HOLES)

CALORIES: 103		FAT: 7g
PROTEIN: 8g		SODIUM: 59mg
FIBER: 2g		CARBOHYDRATES: 13g
NET CARBOHYDRATES: 8g		SUGAR: 1g
SUGAR ALCOHOL: 3g		

HIDDEN CARBS

Be sure to check the labels on protein powders before purchasing. To improve flavor, some brands load up the powders with enough sugar to kick you out of ketosis. Try to avoid any varieties that have more than 4g net carbs per serving. You can also use unflavored whey protein powder in baking.

Chocolate Soufflés

This is one of the simplest desserts you'll ever make, and you'll be glad you did. This recipe will remind you of a mug cake that is ultralight, like a chocolate cloud. It pairs well with a tablespoon of fresh whipped cream and strawberries.

- **Pantry Staples: Coconut oil, vanilla extract**
- **Hands-On Time: 5 minutes**
- **Cook Time: 15 minutes**

Serves 2

- 2 large eggs, whites and yolks separated
- 1 teaspoon vanilla extract
- 2 ounces low-carb chocolate chips
- 2 teaspoons coconut oil, melted

1 In a medium bowl, beat egg whites until stiff peaks form, about 2 minutes. Set aside. In a separate medium bowl, whisk egg yolks and vanilla together. Set aside.

2 In a separate medium microwave-safe bowl, place chocolate chips and drizzle with coconut oil. Microwave on high 20 seconds, then stir and continue cooking in 10-second increments until melted, being careful not to overheat chocolate. Let cool 1 minute.

3 Slowly pour melted chocolate into egg yolks and whisk until smooth. Then, slowly begin adding egg white mixture to chocolate mixture, about ¼ cup at a time, folding in gently.

4 Pour mixture into two 4″ ramekins greased with cooking spray. Place ramekins into air fryer basket. Adjust the temperature to 400°F and set the timer for 15 minutes. Soufflés will puff up while cooking and deflate a little once cooled. The center will be set when done. Let cool 10 minutes, then serve warm.

PER SERVING

CALORIES: 217	**FAT:** 18g
PROTEIN: 8g	**SODIUM:** 71mg
FIBER: 8g	**CARBOHYDRATES:** 19g
NET CARBOHYDRATES: 5g	**SUGAR:** 0g
SUGAR ALCOHOL: 6g	

Chocolate Lava Cakes

This comforting dessert is the perfect treat for chocolate lovers. The chocolate chips provide enough sweetness that you don't need additional sweetener. Try pairing with a scoop of low-carb ice cream such as Rebel for an indulgent goodie that won't get you off track.

- **Pantry Staples: Vanilla extract**
- **Hands-On Time: 5 minutes**
- **Cook Time: 15 minutes**

Serves 2

2 large eggs, whisked

¼ cup blanched finely ground almond flour

½ teaspoon vanilla extract

2 ounces low-carb chocolate chips, melted

1 In a medium bowl, mix eggs with flour and vanilla. Fold in chocolate until fully combined.

2 Pour batter into two 4″ ramekins greased with cooking spray. Place ramekins into air fryer basket. Adjust the temperature to 320°F and set the timer for 15 minutes. Cakes will be set at the edges and firm in the center when done. Let cool 5 minutes before serving.

PER SERVING

CALORIES: 260
PROTEIN: 11g
FIBER: 10g
NET CARBOHYDRATES: 5g
SUGAR ALCOHOL: 6g

FAT: 21g
SODIUM: 71mg
CARBOHYDRATES: 21g
SUGAR: 1g

Chilled Strawberry Pie

This pie is fluffy, and the hint of tartness from the sour cream makes a perfect pair with the crispy pecan crust. Be sure to plan ahead to let the no-bake strawberry filling set after cooking.

- Pantry Staples: None
- Hands-On Time: 15 minutes
- Cook Time: 10 minutes

Serves 6

1½ cups whole shelled pecans
1 tablespoon unsalted butter, softened
1 cup heavy whipping cream
12 medium fresh strawberries, hulled
2 tablespoons sour cream

1 Place pecans and butter into a food processor and pulse ten times until a dough forms. Press dough into the bottom of an ungreased 6″ round nonstick baking dish.

2 Place dish into air fryer basket. Adjust the temperature to 320°F and set the timer for 10 minutes. Crust will be firm and golden when done. Let cool 20 minutes.

3 In a large bowl, whisk cream until fluffy and doubled in size, about 2 minutes.

4 In a separate large bowl, mash strawberries until mostly liquid. Fold strawberries and sour cream into whipped cream.

5 Spoon mixture into cooled crust, cover, and place into refrigerator for at least 30 minutes to set. Serve chilled.

PER SERVING

CALORIES: 340
PROTEIN: 3g
FIBER: 3g
NET CARBOHYDRATES: 4g

FAT: 33g
SODIUM: 17mg
CARBOHYDRATES: 7g
SUGAR: 3g

Pumpkin Pie-Spiced Pork Rinds

While it may sound strange, pork rinds make a great sweet snack too! Make this recipe part of a snack mix by letting the rinds cool for 10 minutes, then mixing them in a bowl with low-carb chocolate chips and roasted nuts.

- **Pantry Staples: None**
- **Hands-On Time: 5 minutes**
- **Cook Time: 5 minutes**

Serves 4

3 ounces plain pork rinds

2 tablespoons salted butter, melted

1 teaspoon pumpkin pie spice

¼ cup confectioners' erythritol

AIR FRYERS AND ERYTHRITOL
When not baked into something, erythritol can quickly begin smoking in the high temperatures of the air fryer. Remember to add the erythritol in this recipe *after* cooking is completed to avoid burning.

1 In a large bowl, toss pork rinds in butter. Sprinkle with pumpkin pie spice, then toss to evenly coat.

2 Place pork rinds into ungreased air fryer basket. Adjust the temperature to 400°F and set the timer for 5 minutes. Pork rinds will be golden when done.

3 Transfer rinds to a medium serving bowl and sprinkle with erythritol. Serve immediately.

PER SERVING

CALORIES: 173	FAT: 13g
PROTEIN: 12g	SODIUM: 394mg
FIBER: 0g	CARBOHYDRATES: 9g
NET CARBOHYDRATES: 0g	SUGAR: 0g
SUGAR ALCOHOL: 9g	

Brown Sugar Cookies

Brown erythritol is the low-carb equivalent of brown sugar. You can find it made by brands like Swerve and Lakanto. It's deeper in flavor than regular sugar, which makes it perfect for sugar cookies. If it isn't readily available to you, you can also use regular granular erythritol with an extra ½ teaspoon vanilla.

- **Pantry Staples: Baking powder, vanilla extract**
- **Hands-On Time: 5 minutes**
- **Cook Time: 27 minutes**

Yields 9 cookies

4 tablespoons salted butter, melted

⅓ cup granular brown erythritol

1 large egg

½ teaspoon vanilla extract

1 cup blanched finely ground almond flour

½ teaspoon baking powder

1 In a large bowl, whisk together butter, erythritol, egg, and vanilla. Add flour and baking powder, and stir until combined.

2 Separate dough into nine pieces and roll into balls, about 2 tablespoons each.

3 Cut three pieces of parchment paper to fit your air fryer basket and place three cookies on each ungreased piece. Place one piece of parchment into air fryer basket. Adjust the temperature to 300°F and set the timer for 9 minutes. Edges of cookies will be browned when done. Repeat with remaining cookies. Serve warm.

PER SERVING (1 COOKIE)

CALORIES: 129		**FAT:** 12g
PROTEIN: 3g		**SODIUM:** 75mg
FIBER: 1g		**CARBOHYDRATES:** 9g
NET CARBOHYDRATES: 1g		**SUGAR:** 1g
SUGAR ALCOHOL: 7g		

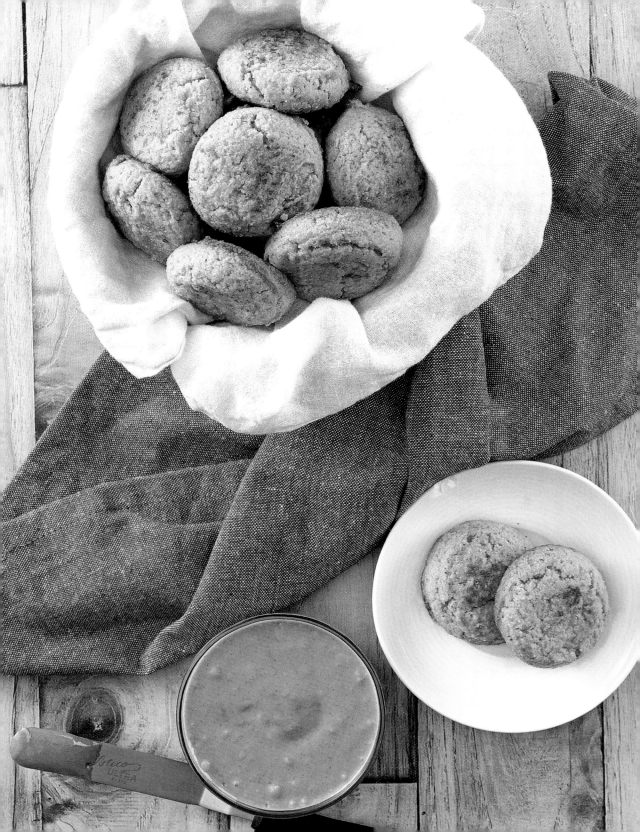

Peanut Butter Cookies

This is a great staple recipe for those peanut butter lovers. It has a strong peanut butter taste without using a large amount. Feel free to swap for no-sugar-added almond butter if you prefer.

- **Pantry Staples: Baking powder, vanilla extract**
- **Hands-On Time: 5 minutes**
- **Cook Time: 27 minutes**

Yields 9 cookies

2 tablespoons salted butter, melted

2 tablespoons all-natural, no-sugar-added peanut butter

⅓ cup granular brown erythritol

1 large egg

½ teaspoon vanilla extract

1 cup blanched finely ground almond flour

½ teaspoon baking powder

1 In a large bowl, whisk together butter, peanut butter, erythritol, egg, and vanilla. Add flour and baking powder, and stir until combined.

2 Separate dough into nine equal pieces and roll each into a ball, about 2 tablespoons each.

3 Cut three pieces of parchment to fit your air fryer basket and place three cookies on each ungreased piece.

4 Place one piece of parchment with cookies into air fryer basket. Adjust the temperature to 300°F and set the timer for 9 minutes. Edges of cookies will be browned when done. Repeat with remaining cookies. Serve warm.

PER SERVING (1 COOKIE)

CALORIES: 129	FAT: 11g
PROTEIN: 4g	SODIUM: 55mg
FIBER: 2g	CARBOHYDRATES: 10g
NET CARBOHYDRATES: 1g	SUGAR: 1g
SUGAR ALCOHOL: 7g	

ALL-NATURAL PEANUT BUTTER

Be sure to check labels to avoid any products with added sugar. Peanuts naturally have 1g–2g sugar per serving; any more than that may have been added during processing. Some stores may also have grind-your-own peanut butter.

Chocolate Chip Cookie Cake

This mini cookie cake is perfect for everything from a small birthday celebration to a simple craving for sweets. The chewy texture is just like a bakery-fresh cookie, but it's made in a fraction of the time!

- **Pantry Staples: Baking powder, vanilla extract**
- **Hands-On Time: 5 minutes**
- **Cook Time: 15 minutes**

Serves 8

4 tablespoons salted butter, melted

⅓ cup granular brown erythritol

1 large egg

½ teaspoon vanilla extract

1 cup blanched finely ground almond flour

½ teaspoon baking powder

¼ cup low-carb chocolate chips

1 In a large bowl, whisk together butter, erythritol, egg, and vanilla. Add flour and baking powder, and stir until combined.

2 Fold in chocolate chips, then spoon batter into an ungreased 6" round nonstick baking dish.

3 Place dish into air fryer basket. Adjust the temperature to 300°F and set the timer for 15 minutes. When edges are browned, cookie cake will be done.

4 Slice and serve warm.

PER SERVING

CALORIES: 170	FAT: 16g
PROTEIN: 4g	SODIUM: 84mg
FIBER: 4g	CARBOHYDRATES: 15g
NET CARBOHYDRATES: 4g	SUGAR: 1g
SUGAR ALCOHOL: 7g	

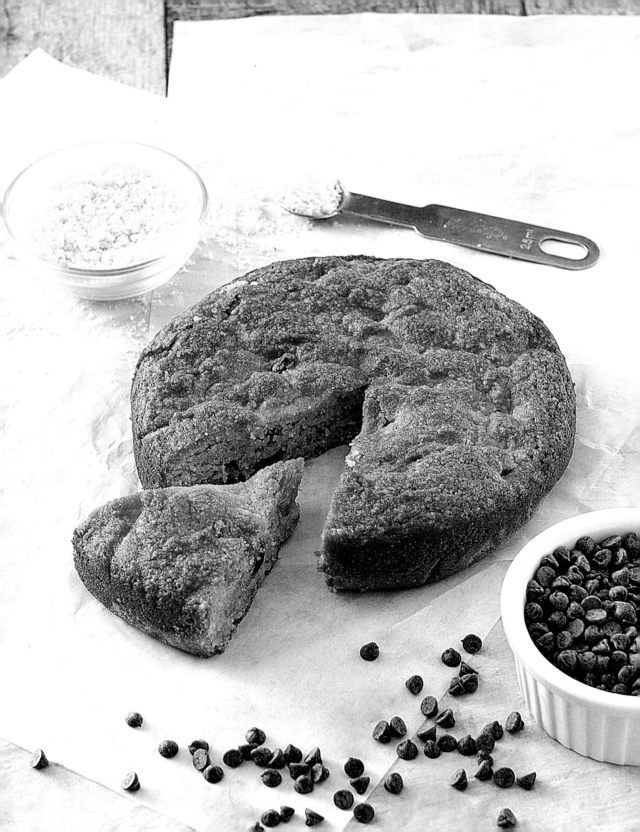

Olive Oil Cake

This is a unique and delicate cake for those who love the mild flavor of olive oil. You'll want to grab a quality bottle for this recipe because the taste will set the tone for the cake. Add a tablespoon of fresh whipped cream to serve.

- **Pantry Staples: Baking powder, vanilla extract**
- **Hands-On Time: 10 minutes**
- **Cook Time: 30 minutes**

Serves 8

2 cups blanched finely ground almond flour
5 large eggs, whisked
¾ cup extra-virgin olive oil
⅓ cup granular erythritol
1 teaspoon vanilla extract
1 teaspoon baking powder

EXTRA-VIRGIN OLIVE OIL

This is the time to pull out your best olive oil. Extra-virgin is unrefined and less processed than the cheaper olive oils used for everyday cooking. Your cake will taste like the oil you use, so choose a flavor you love.

1 In a large bowl, mix all ingredients. Pour batter into an ungreased 6" round nonstick baking dish.

2 Place dish into air fryer basket. Adjust the temperature to 300°F and set the timer for 30 minutes. The cake will be golden on top and firm in the center when done.

3 Let cake cool in dish 30 minutes before slicing and serving.

PER SERVING

CALORIES: 395	FAT: 37g
PROTEIN: 10g	SODIUM: 105mg
FIBER: 3g	CARBOHYDRATES: 13g
NET CARBOHYDRATES: 2g	SUGAR: 1g
SUGAR ALCOHOL: 8g	

Roasted Pecan Clusters

Roasting nuts has never been easier than with an air fryer. In just minutes they come out crunchy, making this a great dessert when you need a last-minute treat. You can also swap out the pecans for an equal amount of almonds if you prefer.

- **Pantry Staples: None**
- **Hands-On Time: 35 minutes**
- **Cook Time: 8 minutes**

Serves 8

3 ounces whole shelled pecans

1 tablespoon salted butter, melted

2 teaspoons confectioners' erythritol

½ teaspoon ground cinnamon

½ cup low-carb chocolate chips

1 In a medium bowl, toss pecans with butter, then sprinkle with erythritol and cinnamon.

2 Place pecans into ungreased air fryer basket. Adjust the temperature to 350°F and set the timer for 8 minutes, shaking the basket two times during cooking. They will feel soft initially but get crunchy as they cool.

3 Line a large baking sheet with parchment paper.

4 Place chocolate in a medium microwave-safe bowl. Microwave on high, heating in 20-second increments and stirring until melted. Place 1 teaspoon chocolate in a rounded mound on ungreased parchment-lined baking sheet, then press 1 pecan into top, repeating with remaining chocolate and pecans.

5 Place baking sheet into refrigerator to cool at least 30 minutes. Once cooled, store clusters in a large sealed container in refrigerator up to 5 days.

PER SERVING

CALORIES: 136	**FAT:** 13g
PROTEIN: 2g	**SODIUM:** 11mg
FIBER: 5g	**CARBOHYDRATES:** 11g
NET CARBOHYDRATES: 2g	**SUGAR:** 0g
SUGAR ALCOHOL: 4g	

Brownies for Two

Pop these into the air fryer while you're enjoying dinner for a perfectly timed dessert that will have you out of the kitchen in record time. Feel free to customize this recipe with your own brownie favorites, such as chopped nuts or low-carb chocolate chips.

- **Pantry Staples: Baking powder, vanilla extract**
- **Hands-On Time: 5 minutes**
- **Cook Time: 15 minutes**

Serves 2

½ cup blanched finely ground almond flour

3 tablespoons granular erythritol

3 tablespoons unsweetened cocoa powder

½ teaspoon baking powder

1 teaspoon vanilla extract

2 large eggs, whisked

2 tablespoons salted butter, melted

1 In a medium bowl, combine flour, erythritol, cocoa powder, and baking powder.

2 Add in vanilla, eggs, and butter, and stir until a thick batter forms.

3 Pour batter into two 4" ramekins greased with cooking spray and place ramekins into air fryer basket. Adjust the temperature to 325°F and set the timer for 15 minutes. Centers will be firm when done. Let ramekins cool 5 minutes before serving.

PER SERVING

CALORIES: 367	FAT: 31g
PROTEIN: 14g	SODIUM: 285mg
FIBER: 6g	CARBOHYDRATES: 29g
NET CARBOHYDRATES: 5g	SUGAR: 2g
SUGAR ALCOHOL: 18g	

MAKE IT À LA MODE!

There are several keto-friendly ice creams available in your grocery store, but you can also make an easy no-churn ice cream at home by adding 1 cup heavy whipping cream to ½ teaspoon vanilla extract and ½ cup confectioners' erythritol. Whisk ingredients in a large bowl and place in the freezer for 2 hours until semi-firm.

Cinnamon Pretzels

Cheese-based doughs are popular for those on the keto diet because of their versatility. It can be turned into anything from lasagna noodles to pizza, and yes, even pretzels! The sweetened dough and cinnamon mask the cheese to make for a crispy and delicious treat.

- **Pantry Staples: None**
- **Hands-On Time: 10 minutes**
- **Cook Time: 10 minutes**

Serves 6

1½ cups shredded mozzarella cheese

1 cup blanched finely ground almond flour

2 tablespoons salted butter, melted, divided

¼ cup granular erythritol, divided

1 teaspoon ground cinnamon

1 Place mozzarella, flour, 1 tablespoon butter, and 2 tablespoons erythritol in a large microwave-safe bowl. Microwave on high 45 seconds, then stir with a fork until a smooth dough ball forms.

2 Separate dough into six equal sections. Gently roll each section into a 12" rope, then fold into a pretzel shape.

3 Place pretzels into ungreased air fryer basket. Adjust the temperature to 370°F and set the timer for 8 minutes, turning pretzels halfway through cooking.

4 In a small bowl, combine remaining butter, remaining erythritol, and cinnamon. Brush ½ mixture on both sides of pretzels.

5 Place pretzels back into air fryer and cook an additional 2 minutes at 370°F.

6 Transfer pretzels to a large plate. Brush on both sides with remaining butter mixture, then let cool 5 minutes before serving.

PER SERVING

CALORIES: 223	**FAT:** 19g
PROTEIN: 11g	**SODIUM:** 222mg
FIBER: 2g	**CARBOHYDRATES:** 13g
NET CARBOHYDRATES: 3g	**SUGAR:** 1g
SUGAR ALCOHOL: 8g	

Easy Keto Danish

Enjoying a creamy Danish doesn't have to be a thing of the past! This quick and keto-friendly dough turns into a golden dessert that's sure to win your heart. Enjoy with fresh strawberries on the side or a teaspoon of sugar-free raspberry preserves in the center.

- **Pantry Staples: None**
- **Hands-On Time: 10 minutes**
- **Cook Time: 12 minutes**

Serves 6

1½ cups shredded mozzarella cheese

½ cup blanched finely ground almond flour

3 ounces cream cheese, divided

¼ cup confectioners' erythritol

1 tablespoon lemon juice

1. Place mozzarella, flour, and 1 ounce cream cheese in a large microwave-safe bowl. Microwave on high 45 seconds, then stir with a fork until a soft dough forms.

2. Separate dough into six equal sections and press each in a single layer into an ungreased 4″ × 4″ square nonstick baking dish to form six even squares that touch.

3. In a small bowl, mix remaining cream cheese, erythritol, and lemon juice. Place 1 tablespoon mixture in center of each piece of dough in baking dish. Fold all four corners of each dough piece halfway to center to reach cream cheese mixture.

4. Place dish into air fryer. Adjust the temperature to 320°F and set the timer for 12 minutes. The center and edges will be browned when done. Let cool 10 minutes before serving.

PER SERVING

CALORIES: 190	**FAT:** 14g
PROTEIN: 10g	**SODIUM:** 244mg
FIBER: 1g	**CARBOHYDRATES:** 10g
NET CARBOHYDRATES: 3g	**SUGAR:** 1g
SUGAR ALCOHOL: 6g	

Coconut Flour Cake

Coconut flour has a natural sweetness that makes it perfect for baking. You need only about ⅓ of the amount as compared to almond flour, which makes it great for budgeting. This cake is naturally moist and baked into a dark golden-brown top that will wow you!

- **Pantry Staples: Baking powder, vanilla extract**
- **Hands-On Time: 10 minutes**
- **Cook Time: 25 minutes**

Serves 6

2 tablespoons salted butter, melted

⅓ cup coconut flour

2 large eggs, whisked

½ cup granular erythritol

1 teaspoon baking powder

1 teaspoon vanilla extract

½ cup sour cream

1 Mix all ingredients in a large bowl. Pour batter into an ungreased 6″ round nonstick baking dish.

2 Place baking dish into air fryer basket. Adjust the temperature to 300°F and set the timer for 25 minutes. The cake will be dark golden on top, and a toothpick inserted in the center should come out clean when done.

3 Let cool in dish 15 minutes before slicing and serving.

PER SERVING

CALORIES: 123

PROTEIN: 4g

FIBER: 2g

NET CARBOHYDRATES: 3g

SUGAR ALCOHOL: 16g

FAT: 9g

SODIUM: 148mg

CARBOHYDRATES: 21g

SUGAR: 2g

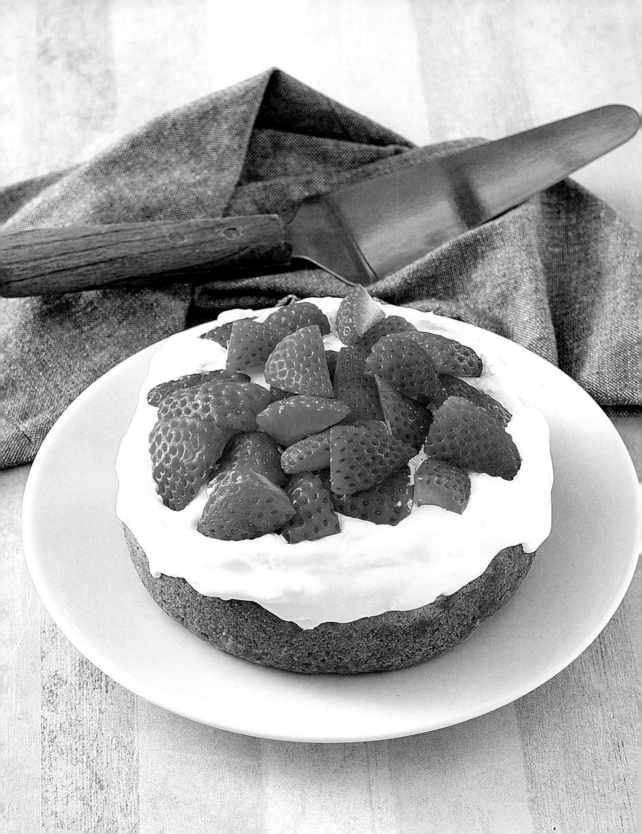

Strawberry Shortcake

This dessert is a keto dream, since whipped cream is naturally low-carb. Whether you're making this for home or a special gathering, it's sure to be a hit!

- **Pantry Staples: Baking powder, coconut oil, vanilla extract**
- **Hands-On Time: 1 hour 10 minutes**
- **Cook Time: 25 minutes**

Serves 6

2 tablespoons coconut oil

1 cup blanched finely ground almond flour

2 large eggs, whisked

½ cup granular erythritol

1 teaspoon baking powder

1 teaspoon vanilla extract

2 cups sugar-free whipped cream

6 medium fresh strawberries, hulled and sliced

1. In a large bowl, combine coconut oil, flour, eggs, erythritol, baking powder, and vanilla. Pour batter into an ungreased 6″ round non-stick baking dish.

2. Place dish into air fryer basket. Adjust the temperature to 300°F and set the timer for 25 minutes. When done, shortcake should be golden and a toothpick inserted in the middle will come out clean.

3. Remove dish from fryer and let cool 1 hour.

4. Once cooled, top cake with whipped cream and strawberries to serve.

PER SERVING

CALORIES: 235	FAT: 21g
PROTEIN: 6g	SODIUM: 104mg
FIBER: 2g	CARBOHYDRATES: 21g
NET CARBOHYDRATES: 3g	SUGAR: 1g
SUGAR ALCOHOL: 16g	

Cream Cheese Shortbread Cookies

These golden, delicious cookies will surprise you with their flavor! They don't taste like cream cheese, but they have a rich, shortbread-like quality. Try adding chopped pecans for a more classic shortbread taste!

- **Pantry Staples: Coconut oil**
- **Hands-On Time: 40 minutes**
- **Cook Time: 20 minutes**

Yields 12 cookies

¼ cup coconut oil, melted

2 ounces cream cheese, softened

½ cup granular erythritol

1 large egg, whisked

2 cups blanched finely ground almond flour

1 teaspoon almond extract

ALMOND EXTRACT

Almond extract is the secret to this recipe's success. It gives the cookie a hint of cherry flavor that reminds you of shortbread. You can swap it for vanilla or even maple extract if preferred.

1 Combine all ingredients in a large bowl to form a firm ball.

2 Place dough on a sheet of plastic wrap and roll into a 12"-long log shape. Roll log in plastic wrap and place in refrigerator 30 minutes to chill.

3 Remove log from plastic and slice into twelve equal cookies. Cut two sheets of parchment paper to fit air fryer basket. Place six cookies on each ungreased sheet. Place one sheet with cookies into air fryer basket. Adjust the temperature to 320°F and set the timer for 10 minutes, turning cookies halfway through cooking. They will be lightly golden when done. Repeat with remaining cookies.

4 Let cool 15 minutes before serving to avoid crumbling.

PER SERVING (1 COOKIE)

CALORIES: 175	**FAT:** 16g
PROTEIN: 5g	**SODIUM:** 23mg
FIBER: 2g	**CARBOHYDRATES:** 12g
NET CARBOHYDRATES: 2g	**SUGAR:** 1g
SUGAR ALCOHOL: 8g	

Pumpkin Cake

This lightly sweet, fluffy cake has warm flavors that would be perfectly complemented by a topping of whipped cream and a sprinkle of cinnamon. Just be sure you purchase pure pumpkin puree and not pumpkin pie filling, which has added sugar!

- **Pantry Staples: Salt, baking powder**
- **Hands-On Time: 10 minutes**
- **Cook Time: 25 minutes**

Serves 8

4 tablespoons salted butter, melted

½ cup granular brown erythritol

¼ cup pure pumpkin puree

1 cup blanched finely ground almond flour

½ teaspoon baking powder

⅛ teaspoon salt

1 teaspoon pumpkin pie spice

EGG-FREE BAKING

That's right, this is an eggless cake! Pumpkin puree can be used in place of eggs (¼ cup puree equals 1 egg) in many baked recipes. Try it out the next time you're running low on eggs.

1 Mix all ingredients in a large bowl. Pour batter into an ungreased 6″ round nonstick baking dish.

2 Place dish into air fryer basket. Adjust the temperature to 300°F and set the timer for 25 minutes. The top will be dark brown, and a toothpick inserted in the center should come out clean when done. Let cool 30 minutes before serving.

PER SERVING

CALORIES: 139	FAT: 13g
PROTEIN: 3g	SODIUM: 112mg
FIBER: 2g	CARBOHYDRATES: 15g
NET CARBOHYDRATES: 1g	SUGAR: 1g
SUGAR ALCOHOL: 12g	

Lime Bars

Limes have a slightly bitter taste, but with a little sweetener they can create a flavorful treat. The buttery crust makes this dessert irresistible and something the whole family will enjoy! Feel free to dust the top with 2 tablespoons confectioners' erythritol before slicing and serving.

- **Pantry Staples: None**
- **Hands-On Time: 10 minutes**
- **Cook Time: 33 minutes**

Yields 12 bars

1½ cups blanched finely ground almond flour, divided

¾ cup confectioners' erythritol, divided

4 tablespoons salted butter, melted

½ cup fresh lime juice

2 large eggs, whisked

1 In a medium bowl, mix together 1 cup flour, ¼ cup erythritol, and butter. Press mixture into bottom of an ungreased 6" round non-stick cake pan.

2 Place pan into air fryer basket. Adjust the temperature to 300°F and set the timer for 13 minutes. Crust will be brown and set in the middle when done.

3 Allow to cool in pan 10 minutes.

4 In a medium bowl, combine remaining flour, remaining erythritol, lime juice, and eggs. Pour mixture over cooled crust and return to air fryer for 20 minutes at 300°F. Top will be browned and firm when done.

5 Let cool completely in pan, about 30 minutes, then chill covered in the refrigerator 1 hour. Serve chilled.

PER SERVING

CALORIES: 133
PROTEIN: 4g
FIBER: 2g
NET CARBOHYDRATES: 1g
SUGAR ALCOHOL: 9g

FAT: 12g
SODIUM: 42mg
CARBOHYDRATES: 12g
SUGAR: 1g

US/Metric Conversion Chart

VOLUME CONVERSIONS

US Volume Measure	Metric Equivalent
⅛ teaspoon	0.5 milliliter
¼ teaspoon	1 milliliter
½ teaspoon	2 milliliters
1 teaspoon	5 milliliters
½ tablespoon	7 milliliters
1 tablespoon (3 teaspoons)	15 milliliters
2 tablespoons (1 fluid ounce)	30 milliliters
¼ cup (4 tablespoons)	60 milliliters
⅓ cup	90 milliliters
½ cup (4 fluid ounces)	125 milliliters
⅔ cup	160 milliliters
¾ cup (6 fluid ounces)	180 milliliters
1 cup (16 tablespoons)	250 milliliters
1 pint (2 cups)	500 milliliters
1 quart (4 cups)	1 liter (about)

WEIGHT CONVERSIONS

US Weight Measure	Metric Equivalent
½ ounce	15 grams
1 ounce	30 grams
2 ounces	60 grams
3 ounces	85 grams
¼ pound (4 ounces)	115 grams
½ pound (8 ounces)	225 grams
¾ pound (12 ounces)	340 grams
1 pound (16 ounces)	454 grams

OVEN TEMPERATURE CONVERSIONS

Degrees Fahrenheit	Degrees Celsius
200 degrees F	95 degrees C
250 degrees F	120 degrees C
275 degrees F	135 degrees C
300 degrees F	150 degrees C
325 degrees F	160 degrees C
350 degrees F	180 degrees C
375 degrees F	190 degrees C
400 degrees F	205 degrees C
425 degrees F	220 degrees C
450 degrees F	230 degrees C

BAKING PAN SIZES

American	Metric
8 x 1½ inch round baking pan	20 x 4 cm cake tin
9 x 1½ inch round baking pan	23 x 3.5 cm cake tin
11 x 7 x 1½ inch baking pan	28 x 18 x 4 cm baking tin
13 x 9 x 2 inch baking pan	30 x 20 x 5 cm baking tin
2 quart rectangular baking dish	30 x 20 x 3 cm baking tin
15 x 10 x 2 inch baking pan	30 x 25 x 2 cm baking tin (Swiss roll tin)
9 inch pie plate	22 x 4 or 23 x 4 cm pie plate
7 or 8 inch springform pan	18 or 20 cm springform or loose bottom cake tin
9 x 5 x 3 inch loaf pan	23 x 13 x 7 cm or 2 lb narrow loaf or pate tin
1½ quart casserole	1.5 liter casserole
2 quart casserole	2 liter casserole

Index

Note: Page numbers in **bold** indicate recipe category lists.

CREATIVE RECIPES

for the Hottest New Kitchen Appliance!

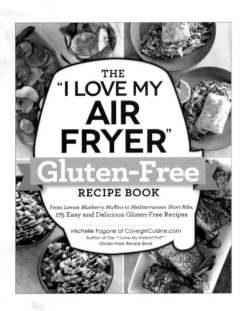
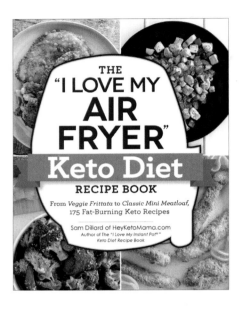
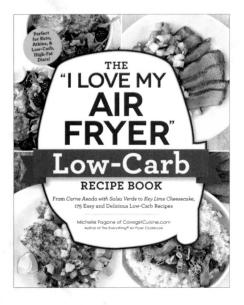
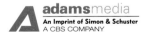